NURSE MANAGERS' BOOKSHELF
A Quarterly Series
VOLUME 2, NUMBER 1, MARCH 1990

Creating an Ethical Environment

The First Century
1890-1990
SANS TACHE

EDITORIAL ADVISORY BOARD

NURSE MANAGERS' BOOKSHELF
A Quarterly Series
VOLUME 2, NUMBER 1, MARCH 1990

Creating an Ethical Environment

JUNE LEVINE-ARIFF, RN, MSN, CNA
Assistant Administrator
Patient Care Services
St. Luke Medical Center
Pasadena, California

DONNA H. GROH, RN, MSN
Director of Nursing
Critical Care Services
Childrens Hospital Los Angeles
Los Angeles, California

WILLIAMS & WILKINS
Baltimore • Hong Kong • London • Sydney

Editor: Susan M. Glover
Associate Editor: Marjorie Kidd Keating
Copy Editor: Shelley Potler
Designer: Norman W. Och
Illustration Planner: Ray Lowman
Production Coordinator: Raymond E. Reter

Williams & Wilkins
428 East Preston Street
Baltimore, Maryland 21202, USA

Printed in the United States of America

Library of Congress Cataloging in Publication Data

Levine-Ariff, June.
Creating an ethical environment / June Levine-Ariff, Donna H. Groh.
p. cm.—(Nurse managers' bookshelf ; v. 2, no. 1 (Mar. 1990))
Includes bibliographical references.
ISBN 0-683-06534-3
1. Nursing ethics. I. Groh, Donna H. II. Title. III. Series: Nurse managers' bookshelf ; v. 2, no. 1.
RT85.L48 1990
174'.2—dc20 89-70436
CIP

90 91 92 93
1 2 3 4 5 6 7 8 9 10

MANAGING EDITOR'S FOREWORD

As we enter the last decade of the 20th century, several of the trends predicted by author John Naisbitt in his best-seller, *Megatrends,* are emerging. How are these trends affecting health care delivery systems and health care providers? And, more important, how can we facilitate our staff's adjustment to, acceptance of, and comfort with these changes, which are sometimes exciting but more often disconcerting, if not downright anxiety provoking? In this second volume of *Nurse Managers' Bookshelf* we provide some answers to these questions, answers that will assist you with the toughest—and most important—part of your job, the PEOPLE PART.

As nursing departments become decentralized, nurse managers are undergoing role changes. Your old role as a boss is giving way to a new role as a coach or advisor; you are deriving more credibility from your managerial expertise than from your clinical competence; you are developing management techniques that encourage employee risk taking and innovative problem solving; and you are giving people the trust that they deserve. Without abdicating your responsibilities as a manager, you have been building relationships and putting issues in proper perspective, recognizing that unpopular decisions are sometimes part of the job.

Recognizing your need to stay informed about emerging issues and the necessity to achieve a broader perspective about the increasingly complex practice environment, the Editorial Advisory Board has chosen ethics, information systems, managerial styles, and problem employee behaviors as topics for this year's volume. These four issues will provide a fresh perspective, stimulate thinking, and cultivate self-esteem as the keys to enhancing employee satisfaction and empowerment, with resulting quality patient care. As always, we would like to hear your thoughts and reactions to these topics and your suggestions for future issues.

Susan M. Glover, RN, MSN
Managing Editor

PREFACE

When we told people we were writing a book on ethics and management, most of them were amused and skeptical that the two concepts would be considered in the same book. Although we all laughed together, the fact is that only recently have these two concepts been openly discussed together in the literature. We also recognize that just as ethics is a new topic in nursing education, the combining of ethical principles and management standards has yet to be fully realized. So, we wrote this book simply because we believe that effective nursing management is based on an ethical commitment to patient care.

An initial discussion about patient advocacy sets the stage for a look into creating environments where ethical decision making can occur. The Code for Nurses and a review of ethical principles form the basis for the chapter on ethical decision making. These chapters establish a framework from which to discuss confronting unsafe practice and whistleblowing. The chapters on institutional mechanisms and policies give guidance to nurse managers who are involved with ethical concerns. Obviously, one of the most critical dilemmas faced by nursing managers is the availability and utilization of registered nurses; this is addressed in the chapter on allocation of nursing resources. Throughout, the text emphasizes the central role played by nursing management in integrating all the components into a whole that will comprise an approach to nursing management that has as its focus the creation of an ethical environment for practice. To avoid redundancy and awkwardness in expression, we have chosen to use the pronouns "she," "her," and "hers" for nurses and nurse managers since 98% of nurses in the United States are female.

We owe special thanks to Andrew Jameton, whose moral support and professional guidance aided us greatly; to Jackie Clark for assistance in manuscript preparation; to our families—Michael and Benjamin, and Marty, Kevin, and Erin—who gave support and encouragement throughout the process; and lastly, to Bonnie Siegal, RN, MN, and the Nursing Department of Childrens Hospital Los Angeles, to whom we extend our appreciation for enabling our growth and supporting our ability to integrate these concepts into practice.

June Levine-Ariff, RN, MSN, CNA
Donna H. Groh, RN, MSN

CONTENTS

Managing Editor's Foreword v
Preface vii

1 Creating an Ethical Environment 1

2 Professional Ethics 17

3 Ethical Decision Making 41

4 Confronting Unsafe Practice 62

5 Whistleblowing 84

6 Institutional Forums 101

7 Ethical Guidelines 121

8 The Allocation of Scarce Nursing Resources 130

Suggested Readings 157

Index 159

1

Creating an Ethical Environment

"It is better to light one candle than curse the darkness"[1] (Blanchard & Peale, 1988). Creating an ethical environment within a bureaucratic structure may at first seem humorous, if not impossible. To create an environment means to apply principles that set the stage for implementing a certain way of thinking and acting. Since ethics concerns itself with doing good, truth telling, promise keeping, respect for persons, and so on, creating an ethical environment means to build these concepts into the usual and customary practices of the organization. Ethics gives people guidelines for what would be morally permissible behavior, but it also stresses individual decision making and allows for flexibility based on individual considerations. When one thinks of the characteristics of bureaucracies, these are not the precepts that may immediately come to mind. In fact, it frequently seems more difficult to act ethically within a bureaucratic structure than in other environments.

Bureaucracies often act in strange ways and perpetuate ritualistic behavior. Bureaucratic structures evolve within organizations both small and large. Sometimes, they seem to feed on themselves. New programs and new regulations give rise to new departments and more layers of hierarchy. Political factors and professional lines of territoriality play a role in the development of the bureaucracy. Due to the numbers of people in various positions, the large number of external commitments, and the unwritten rules that spring up, written policies and procedures are developed to tell people how they are expected to behave in certain situations. In fact, that is also what ethics does—provide guidance about how one should behave in certain circumstances. But procedures and policies give us a structured way to act by asking that we do specific things in a specific way. Ethics, on the other hand, asks that we adhere to specific concepts and fosters a belief in an individual's autonomous ability to make decisions and act accordingly. It is here that we begin to anticipate some potential conflict in being able to act ethically within a bureaucratic organization, if the rules developed by the bureaucracy are inflexible and incongruent with ethical standards.

Ethics has always been an integral part of clinical nursing practice. From its inception as a professional group, nursing has been concerned with the moral responsibility of its practitioners, has expressed a commitment to high ideals for providing service, and has professed a belief in the central role that nurses play in the improvement of patient welfare. Nurses are taught that their first responsibility is to the patient. However, nurses work as employees of an institution and thus have some responsibility to the institution that employs them. This can cause conflict for a nurse. When nurses enter the work world of an organization, they find the work environment usually quite structured. Adherence to policies and procedures and a bureaucratic hierarchy supercede an educational thrust that reinforced autonomous decision making and individualized patient care. The role expectations of the workplace seem to be antithetical to the role expectations students learned in school.

As professionals, nurses may experience a strong conflict between what they think ought to be done and what they are expected to do. The profession of nursing asks the nurse to practice according to a code of ethics; however, as employees, nurses are obliged to abide by institutional policies, rules, and expectations. A bureaucracy can intensify the role conflicts nurses face in practice. The demands made by the employing organization often affect the ethical choices nurses make (Yarling & McElmurray, 1986). Organizations that stifle professional autonomy, that favor policies consistent with the good of others rather than patients, and that do not provide for dispute resolution may prevent nurses from acting in a morally autonomous fashion.

Advocacy

Central to the Code for Nurses is a recognition of nursing's primary role as a patient advocate. The registered nurse is often the first person to recognize situations that are not in the best interest of the patient; she can either initiate action or report these situations to persons who can effect change. Acts such as these have been termed "patient advocacy"; however, it is important not to confuse the concept of advocacy with the expected practice of every registered nurse. Questioning orders that seem to be inadequate, unclear, or inaccurate is what the nurse is supposed to do. The situation *could* turn into an act of advocacy, should a patient be placed in a potentially harmful situation. For example, a nurse who goes into a patient's room to get a surgical consent form signed is fulfilling her professional responsibility by ascertaining the patient's knowledge about the impending surgery. If the patient were to ask questions or make statements that clearly demonstrated a significant lack of knowledge, the nurse would be fulfilling a professional duty by not having the patient sign the consent and contacting the physician. Acting responsibly, the physician should clear up the patient's misconceptions. The nurse would then get the consent signed, and surgery would proceed. On the other hand, should the physician tell the nurse that he already told the patient what was necessary, that he would not see the patient, and that he wanted the consent signed now, the nurse could certainly find herself in a potential advocacy position. The patient is being denied the truth and does not know it.

The classic definition of advocacy is the act of defending or pleading the case of another. This definition could be applicable to a courtroom situation, when the individual may not be able to act in his/her own behalf. Mary Kohnke offers a definition of advocacy that can be applied to nursing: "Advocacy is the act of informing and supporting a person so that he can make the best decisions possible for himself" (Kohnke, 1988). Thus the nurse must ensure that the patient has all the information he would need to make an informed decision. Then, no matter what the choice, the nurse is there to support the patient. The discussion in Chapter 2, under the principle of autonomy, defines the concept of patient autonomy and the doctrine of informed consent.

For healthcare providers in general, advocacy can be very difficult. It is almost in direct conflict with the image of themselves as people who know best, experts who are paid to know and to make decisions based on their knowledge. As one physician related to this author, " They (patients) pay me to tell them what to do" (personal communication, April 1989). Advocacy is not acting on behalf of someone else. It is assisting patients so they can make informed choices. Kohnke says clearly that advocates must not put themselves in the position of rescuing, a role more compatible with a paternalistic approach to health care (Kohnke, 1982). The role appropriate for all healthcare professionals is to serve as advisors, sharing their specific information and certainly offering their recommendations to enable patients to make their own decisions. That is what the patient is really buying. It may be necessary to discuss the issues with the patient on more than one occasion, until the patient can reach his own decision. Finally, it may be necessary to serve as advocates for patients, should a decision by someone else truly not be in the best interest of the patient.

Contrary to some managers' and employees' beliefs, the advocacy role is not incompatible with the role of employee. In fact, most health-care professionals and institutions wish to act in the best interests of their patients. However, the functions of the advocate can, at times, be at odds with the institution's cultural norms. Some institutions give lip service to patient rights. The physician may be quite powerful in the organization, and the nurse, knowing the patient should be told the truth, may find herself blocked and/or admonished for taking on the role of the advocate. Consistent with the discussions on confronting unsafe practice and whistleblowing in later chapters, the advocate must have an understanding about why something is the right thing to do and clarity about the best way to proceed. "Ignorance is the greatest weapon of tyrants and the greatest defense of people who do not want to accept responsibility for themselves" (Kohnke, 1980, p. 2040). There is no doubt that although an individual nurse may act as an advocate for the patient, there will be other nurses and doctors who will be uncomfortable being challenged by their patients. An individual nurse may get pressure to conform to institutional norms about how nurses and patients should act. Thus it behooves any nurse involved in an advocacy situation to recognize, as appropriate, the ethical issues involved and approach ethical decision making in a deliberate manner. To take on the role of patient advocate requires strict adherence to the principles and concepts that guide decision making. It requires a broad knowledge base from which to act.

Historically, the concept of advocacy has been and is an integral part of the nursing profession. In the history of the Code for Nurses, outlined in Chapter 2, it is clear that nurses have always believed that advocating for patients was inherent in their role. In the early years of the profession, advocacy was carried out by adhering to institutional rules and physician orders. Obedience was believed to be the best way to carry out the care the patient ought to receive. As nurses have come to learn, not only was that stance not patient advocacy, but it often worked against such a role. With loyalty as a key virtue, criticism of the institution or the physician was not allowed. Obedience was valued, and so the nurse did not question those in authority. Yet as early as 1910, an editorial appeared in the *American Journal of Nursing* entitled "Where Does Loyalty End?" asking the question, "Is a nurse required to be untruthful or practice deceit to uphold the reputation of the physician at her own expense or that of her patient?"

Loyalty became a dominant theme in early nursing literature. For example, nurses were asked not to tell patients information about their illness, nurses were asked to tell patients that the physician could not be reached (when, in fact, he had spoken with the nurse), nurses were asked not to tell patients why they were receiving certain drugs or getting certain treatments. All this lying caused great conflict within many nurses and perpetuated many questions as to what was the right thing to do in these situations.

While there was an early awareness that the nurse owed the community a larger loyalty than she owed another nurse, this same awareness, unfortunately, did not extend to the physician or institution for many years. "The Tentative Code for the Nursing Profession," presented in 1940, continued to emphasize clear loyalty to the physician, "leaving precious little time for advocacy" (Nelson, 1988). Winslow (1984) believed that the early 1970s was the beginning of significant changes within the profession. However, in Murphy's study (1983) of nurses' moral reasoning during this time period, unquestioning loyalty to the physician and hospital still continued to be a dominant theme for nurses' decision making.

The rise of consumerism, feminism, and a general societal questioning of healthcare costs and the physician's elitist role within society have helped frame the context in which nurses practice currently. The 1985 version of the Code for Nurses clearly affirms the centrality of the role of patient advocate in the profession. It has become clear that the nurse's duty to the patient surpasses loyalty to the physician and the institution where the nurse works. "Nursing Victorian values of unthinking obedience to authority figures and fixed rules and regulations are dysfunctional for the new role of the nurse as a morally responsible agent who is an advocate for the patient and guardian of his right" (Bandman & Bandman, 1978, p. 314).

Risk Versus Duty

Generally, when intervention will meet patient needs, prevent harm, and do good, there is a general duty toward advocacy. In some situations and/or in some institutions, advocacy could imply risk for the nurse. The duty to advocate depends on the level of risk to the nurse. When risk is great but can be reduced, there is an obligation to advocate. When risk cannot be reduced, and the nurse could be significantly harmed, the risk does not have to be taken. "Accepting personal risk which exceeds the limits of duty is not morally obligatory" (American Nurses' Association Committee on Ethics, 1986). The American Nurses' Association's (ANA) statement regarding risk versus responsibility gives some guidance as to when risk implies a moral duty versus a moral option:

1) The patient is at significant risk of harm or damage if the nurse does not assist.
2) The nurse's intervention or care is directly relevant to preventing harm.
3) The nurse's care will probably prevent harm, loss, or damage to the patient.
4) The benefit the patient will gain outweighs any harm the nurse might incur and does not present more than minimal risk to the health care provider. (American Nurses' Association Committee on Ethics, 1986).

The degree of risk to the nurse in situations of advocacy is influenced by the organizational culture and norms. A situation may pose significant risk for an individual in one environment, while the identical situation in a different institution with different norms would carry no risk at all. In fact, the scenario may not even arise as a situation of advocacy. Managers encounter situations in which they must advocate for a whole class of patients, or for the nursing staff, or in situations of potential harm to a group of unknown individuals. How risky would these following situations be in your institution?

- The institution has always charged a fee for continuous pulse oximetry monitoring. However, in the intensive care unit (ICU), this noninvasive monitoring technique has been incorporated into the bedside monitors and has become as ubiquitous as cardiorespiratory monitoring, which is not billed as an individual item. The manager feels this service should be viewed as part of the basic ICU accommodations, but dropping the individual charge will mean a decrease of $500,000.00 of potential revenue for the institution. The manager feels strongly that this charge is not ethically justified and decides to push the issue.
- The ICU has a 20% staff nurse vacancy rate. The census has been running very high, and staff have been doing large amounts of overtime. The nurse manager feels she has exhausted all her resources for supplemental staff. The operating room schedule for the next few days is very heavy. The nurse manager does not think those patients

can be handled safely and wants to ask that some elective cases be postponed.

How would you approach these situations in your institution, and what might some of the potential risks and outcomes be?

- You discover kickbacks are being made for the purchase of certain supplies.
- You disagree with a physician who is demanding that a nurse be fired.
- The institutional system demands that all nursing documentation forms be approved by medical staff.

Accountability

Any discussion of advocacy would not be complete without touching on the concept of accountability. The term "advocacy" implies action. To act ethically is better than simply to believe that ethical behavior is good. To be accountable means to be willing to seize responsibility, not wait until it is thrust upon you. This concept highlights the importance of the manager's role. To be accountable for acts of advocacy, one needs an environment that demands and facilitates such action. Unfortunately,

> Nurses seem to be psychologically geared to respond to others rather than to initiate action. The physician writes the order, the nurse carries it out. The patient rings his bell, the nurse answers it. Perhaps because of this fairly typical sequence of events, nurses have developed a patterned approach to patient care that is almost akin to a conditioned response. (McClure, 1978)

Effective management strategies that promote an ethical environment must build on the nurse's professional socialization, learned in school. Knowing what is the right thing to do and doing it must not end when professionals leave the halls of learning and enter the world of service.

It would be discouraging if the profession of nursing supported Abrams' statement: "Owing to potential conflicts with the nursing hierarchy, the possibility of loss of job or benefit as a result of disobedience in certain situations, the nurse may not be the appropriate person to represent or defend the rights or best interests of a patient" (Abrams, 1978). There is no doubt that institutional loyalties have conflicted with nurses' duty toward patient advocacy. However, Florence Nightingale began a long tradition of patient advocacy when she took action to improve the care the wounded soldiers received during the Crimean War. It was certainly an act of advocacy, and it certainly conflicted with institutional expectations. Because advocacy fits so well with nursing's traditional concern for the health and welfare of patients, the role of patient advocate persists.

The turmoil and conflict faced by many nurses as they enter into advocacy situations are still all too common. What can the profession do to resolve such issues? As the rest of this chapter and subsequent chapters will demonstrate, nursing professionals in management roles can do a lot to relieve the turmoil and conflict by creating an environment in which advocacy is recognized, valued, and supported.

Corporate Culture

The tone for an ethical environment is set by the corporate culture of the institution. Recently, there has been a lot of attention paid to the impact of corporate culture on the overall effectiveness of an organization. According to del Bueno and Vincent (1986), corporate culture is a recent theory that "is a symbolic or cultural view that emphasizes the importance of shared values and norms rather than the structural or rationale variables stressed in traditional theories" about management. Peters and Waterman (1983) certainly found that the notion of shared values and a clear understanding of common goals were critical to the success of organizations. Actions are influenced, indeed determined, by values. If an institution is not clear about what it values, then its employees will have only their individual values to guide their actions. These individual values, while neither right nor wrong, may differ significantly from the values of others in the organization, which will contribute to confusions about what constitutes appropriate behavior.

In writing about obligations to patients, MacNeil states, "It is necessary to have a clear mission statement...because it is essential for the institution to understand why it exists, to understand what it stands for" (1966). A mission statement should embody the organization's commitment to the community and patients it serves. Additionally, organizations create a culture of values related to how people work together, how problem solving is approached, and how situations of conflict are resolved. Not only must the organization define what it stands for and what it values, but this must be clearly communicated to all the individuals who work there. Once those values and that mission have been defined and communicated, it becomes easier for individual practitioners to determine if a particular institution's values are congruent with their own.

The values that are articulated need to be real, not just words that receive lip service. Actions must be congruent with the stated values. It becomes a sham for an institution to claim to value patient autonomy but then allow situations to exist where nurses, who advocate for patients to receive informed consent, can be verbally abused by irate physicians. It can indeed be a soul-searching experience for an institution to come to grips with what it says it values and what behavior actually gets rewarded. Managers must be willing to bring examples of incongruent behavior to the attention of administration. Too often, administrators assume that just because they have published a mission statement or articulated a set of "shared values," everyone throughout the organization is automatically behaving that way. Organizations are always influenced by new individuals and changing times. For an organization's mission to stay current and alive, it must be periodically reviewed and constantly restated, both verbally and through the programs and services the institution is providing. Operationalizing these concepts is frequently easier said than done.

Nursing Philosophy

Creating an environment where ethical practice can thrive also depends on developing a nursing philosophy that clearly defines the responsibility of the individual practitioner and the department of nursing. These responsibilities must incorporate an ethical focus for practice that is accepted and achievable. The department's beliefs about the role of the nurse, its beliefs about the actual role of the department in supporting and operationalizing those concepts must be clearly defined. These beliefs must be congruent with the overall mission of the organization. If they are not, nurse managers and staff will encounter even more conflicts at the bedside and unit level. In situations where nursing's mission and the organization's mission differ, one or both need to be reevaluated.

As in any organization, the ideal can be drowned out by practical realities. It is incumbent upon nursing management to ensure an environment that rises above the noise of reality. A nursing philosophy must be part of daily practice for every nurse in the institution. A philosophy cannot be written and filed away, only to be pulled out when the Joint Commission for Accreditation of Healthcare Organizations (JCAHO) visits. It must be incorporated into the standards of care, the job descriptions, and performance appraisals. The philosophy should be featured in recruitment brochures, and it should be introduced to every new staff nurse at the time of hire and/or orientation to the work setting. What is said about what the department of nursing values sets the stage for how employees interpret their roles. An orientation full of procedures and policies versus a discussion of philosophy and values will give very different messages about what the department expects.

Every project undertaken by the department should be examined to ensure that it is congruent with the philosophy and in some way furthers the department's efforts to make the philosophy a living reality. Every committee or council should have a purpose that supports some aspect of the philosophy, and annual goals and objectives must be reviewed to ensure that they are consistent with carrying out the philosophy. It is only when expectations are translated into action that the possibility for change occurs.

A study by Ketefian (1985) suggested that those individuals with high moral behavior adhere more to professional values, as described by Kramer (loyalty to the nursing profession, involvement in professional organizations, commitment to practice standards and scientific knowledge as the basis for practice) (1968). A philosophy that emphasizes these values would certainly encourage the development of an ethical environment. However, Kramer's research found that baccalaureate graduates change from a professional values orientation to a bureaucratic orientation after they have been fully oriented into the work setting (1974). This finding emphasizes the importance of setting the tone from the outset. Since staff nurses are placed in a role that requires obligations to many different constituencies, it is up to the nurse manager to facilitate an environment where these values are upheld. The young staff nurse must be helped to negotiate the bureaucracy to effectively advocate for patients. The staff nurse must recognize that the nurse manager is there to support this end.

Obligations of the Nurse Manager

It is the nurse manager's responsibility to facilitate a safe and ethical practice environment. From a review of the Code for Nurses, it is clear that managers have an obligation to do the following:

- Provide a safe environment for patients
- Intervene and/or report the illegal or unethical practice of any person
- Ensure privacy and confidentiality of patients
- Ensure an environment for patient advocacy
- Maintain conditions of employment conducive to a quality practice environment
- Ensure privacy and confidentiality of nursing staff

- Ensure a competent nursing staff
- Support and encourage nurses to maintain competence in nursing
- Support the development of policies that foster ethical behavior
- Support the welfare of the nursing profession
- Maintain the integrity of nursing
- Support policies of the hospital and the department of nursing
- Use and encourage the use of organizational channels
- Ensure availability of needed supplies and equipment
- Ensure mechanisms to facilitate delivery of nursing services

The nurse manager must recognize that by providing such an environment, issues the staff may present could challenge tradition, but continuing discussion about ethical issues is absolutely critical to prevent premature and subjective decision. Answering ethical questions does not always produce right answers or wrong answers. Often, it is the consequences of an act, the benefits and burdens, if you will, that determine the outcome. Nurses must be helped down this decision path.

For individuals to act morally, they first must be given the freedom to do so. Knowledge without the mechanism to apply it makes for unhappy and dissatisfied personnel. When a dilemma arises, nurses should be encouraged to use established channels of communication. The nursing staff must have a clear understanding of what those channels are, both within the nursing department and outside it. Staff must know they will be supported if they access those channels in order to follow up on concerns, without having to check it out with the nurse manager first. As needed, the nurse manager can pave the way for the nurse to get the necessary input and support and help the nurse present the concern in a reasoned, logical manner, minimizing emotional or reactional tone. The model for ethical decision making presented in Chapter 3 can be used to assist the nurse in acquiring adequate and appropriate information.

Discussions about decision making options will help the nurse to see various alternatives. Swider, McElmurry, and Yarling (1985) classified student nurses' responses to a hypothetical ethical dilemma. Analysis revealed four response groupings: patient centered, physician centered, bureaucratic centered, and collective action centered. Whether a nurse would choose to tell a patient directly about receiving a wrong medication (patient centered) or go to the supervisor (bureaucratic centered) can help the manager understand how the staff is making decisions. Managers who are not skilled in facilitating this type of discussion should seek other resources (see Chapter 7) to assist them in providing the staff with appropriate consultations.

Setting the Stage

Nursing managers should explore the topic of advocacy at the time of the hiring interview. The nurse manager might give the interviewee a hypothetical situation that would require the nurse to act as a patient advocate. The manager should be inquiring about the nurse's philosophy. What does she see as her primary obligation—carrying out physicians' orders or meeting patients' needs? How does she make decisions and utilize resources? Expectations of the nurse should be delineated. The hospital's mission and the nursing department's philosophy should be shared and explained. By exploring these topics before hiring staff, the nurse manager can discern individuals whose values and professional behavior are congruent with the practice environment the manager is attempting to create.

Likewise, nurses should learn what questions to ask in order to assess an environment supportive of professional practice, which certainly includes the advocacy role. Questions about the nursing philosophy—where it is, what it says, how it is actualized in practice—are good starting points. The nurse might give the interviewer a hypothetical case that would reveal the manager's attitude toward the advocacy role. The nurse should find out whether the department of nursing is actively involved in medical staff and hospital committees. Who represents the nursing department on these committees? Are staff nurses involved with setting direction for the nursing department? What is the procedure when a nurse disagrees with a physician's order?

These questions are not just for the staff nurse looking for a job. They are also questions that can be asked by the nurse manager looking for a management position. For the manager, the answers become critical indicators of her ability to be both a patient and nurse advocate. Questions should be asked about how the institution fulfills its obligations to patients and professional nursing staff, both deserving of autonomy. Interviewing one's prospective employer about whether patient autonomy and nursing advocacy are valued may help an individual avoid employment in nonsupportive environments. At a time when nursing staffing is so critical, nurses can make a statement about the need for professional environments by not working at institutions that impede patient advocacy and thus limit the full actualization of the role of professional nurse.

Leadership and Creativity

Facilitating an ethical environment requires leadership, to take the initiative, to ask questions, and to incorporate the answers into the business of delivering patient care. The environment created by management must stimulate problem solving and foster creativity. It must encourage new and better solutions to old problems. Change must be accepted and desired.

Leadership is not optional, it is essential—for motivation and direction of staff. It is the single most essential ingredient in any organization. Replacing a leader in an organization with a nonleader takes away the vision, the very spirit, of the organization. Employees who once dedicated themselves to that vision begin to drift without leadership.

Managers are not always leaders, and leaders are not always managers. Bennis says that leaders do the right thing, while managers do things right (Research Institute of America, 1985). Ideally, one would be a good leader with sound managerial traits as well. Leaders are goal oriented and willing to take calculated risks to accomplish those goals. They are constantly planning based on future needs. Leaders are flexible in how they approach problems and devise solutions, based on the needs of their followers and the situation. Managers tend to be more oriented toward daily events, and their planning is focused on specific incidents. They are more structured in their approach to situations and tend to be reactive rather than proactive. Leaders are able to inspire and motivate. Managers are able to implement plans. As Lane Longfellow (personal communication, 1988) said, "Martin Luther King didn't say 'I have a plan,' he said 'I have a dream.'"

Good ethics can foster good leadership and good management. Managers must ask if the way something is done is the way it ought to be done. Is patient care being delivered in the way it ought to be delivered? If the same problem arises over and over again, it is time for sorting out other alternatives. There must be a willingness to try new things, to experiment with new ideas to find what will be successful. Managers must create an environment where all staff can contribute ideas for change and not fear rebuke or ridicule if those ideas do not succeed.

Ethics Education

"Little thought has been spent upon our ethical culture....There is a mystery surrounding the term 'ethics' which causes the average nurse to turn away and wait for another to ask the first question or to make the first demand" (Riddle, 1903). Although this statement was made in 1903, and although progress has certainly occurred, much of it could still be called accurate today. There must be more integration of ethics education into undergraduate and graduate nursing education. Educational institutions teach nurses that they should be patient advocates. Yet they fail to teach nurses how to be patient advocates within a bureaucratic structure.

It would be helpful if they taught nurses how to translate the "ideal of service" ("Suggested Code," 1926) into the reality of working in a service organization. They must teach nurses about the social, political, and environmental forces that may inhibit an ethical posture. Every nurse must understand how to maneuver within an organizational hierarchy and around an often paternalistic approach to patient care. This is certainly an area where schools of nursing could benefit from the experiences of nursing managers. A course designed to discuss the difficult dilemmas faced by nurses in the practice setting, with a reality focus on how to deal with particular situations, would be very helpful. It should be designed to introduce the nurse to the tough ethical decisions faced nearly every day in the workplace.

Schools should be offering courses where the students have preceptors who are practicing professionals, for example, a management course where the student would spend half the semester with a primary nurse to see how she manages a caseload of patients and the remainder of the semester with a nurse manager to see how she manages a nursing unit. Instructors from schools of nursing should be spending time periodically in the practice setting without students, to ensure that they are current. Not only should some of this time be devoted to clinical exposure, but also the instructors should be spending time with a nurse manager to see how she is structuring the environment for practice. Additionally, nursing administrators should be lecturing regularly to students, bringing that reality orientation directly into the classroom. Topics that are particularly relevant for administrators to discuss might include leadership versus management, change theory (with an assignment for the students to implement a change project), analysis of performance evaluation systems, and organizational structure and culture. Certainly, as more and more nurses return to school for their baccalaureate degrees in nursing, the profession has a golden opportunity. These individuals are usually motivated to learn, bring the element of experience to the classroom, and are ready to take a constructive leadership approach to care at the bedside.

Summary

It is obvious that institutional structures may pose conflicts as nurses attempt to mediate between organizational culture and norms and professional values. Nurses are constantly being confronted with questions of competing values. Should ability to pay be considered when life-saving technology is available? How can I respect the patient's wishes and not violate institutional policy? Is medical necessity the only indication for admission or continued care in an intensive care unit? What do I do when asked to administer experimental drugs to an uninformed patient? Are the patient's wishes being respected? How do I answer the questions of a competent patient when the physician has asked that the patient not be told the truth?

The position of the nurse manager brings additional competing values into potential conflict. What should the nurse manager do when various staff nurses bring complaints about a specific physician's practice? What should the nurse manager do when the admitting practices of the unit are consistently violated by physicians? What should the nurse manager do when given an inadequate staffing budget, based solely on average census, not on patient acuity? What should the nurse manager do when her request for a piece of equipment vital for patient safety is denied?

The number and variety of ethical dilemmas will only be increasing, not diminishing. It is clear that the nurse manager has additional duties and obligations, beyond those that directly relate to the patient. The nursing staff, the unit, and the institution are also within the scope of the manager's obligation. The nurse manager has the responsibility for establishing systems, policies, and procedures that provide the structure and process to manage these types of issues. As a role model, the nurse manager is in a unique position to influence practices that contribute to an ethical environment. How a nurse manager chooses to enact her role will tell the people she manages what she values. Nurse managers have the moral obligation and responsibility to ensure a climate of ethical advocacy. The fact is that the nursing manager is an advocate for both patients and the nursing staff. The remaining chapters will provide nurse managers with insight, both for themselves and their staffs, as they confront the tough questions that need to be answered.

REFERENCES

Abrams, N. (1978). A contrary view of the nurse as patient advocate. *Nursing Forum, 17*(3), 267.

American Nurses' Association Committee on Ethics. (1986). *Statement regarding risk v. responsibility in providing nursing care.* Kansas City, Mo: American Nurses' Association.

Bandman, E., & Bandman, B. (1978). *Bioethics and human rights.* Boston: Little, Brown.

Blanchard, K., & Peale, N. V. (1988). The power of ethical management. In K.

Blanchard & N. V. Peale (Eds.), *Family partnership* (1st ed., p. 129). New York: William Morrow.
del Bueno, D. J., & Vincent, P. M. (1986). Organizational culture: How important is it? *Journal of Nursing Administration, 16*(10), 15–20.
Ketefian, S. (1985). Professional and bureaucratic role conceptions and moral behavior among nurses. *Nursing Research, 34*(4), 248–253.
Kohnke, M. F. (1982). *Advocacy risk and reality.* St. Louis: C. V. Mosby.
Kohnke, M. F. (1980). The nurse as advocate. *American Journal of Nursing, 88,* 2038–2040.
Kramer, M. (1968). Role models, role conceptions, and role deprivation. *Nursing Research, 17,* 115–120.
Kramer, M. (1974). Reality shock: Why nurses leave nursing. St. Louis: C. V. Mosby.
MacNeil, E. (1986). The responsibility of the organization to the patient/resident. *CHAC Review, 14*(4), 4–7.
McClure, M. L. (1978). The long road to accountability. *Nursing Outlook, Jan.,* 47–50.
Murphy, C. P. (1983). Models of the nurse-patient relationship. In C. P. Murphy & H. Hunter (Eds.), *Ethical problems in the nurse-patient relationship* (pp. 8–24). New York: Allyn & Bacon.
Nelson, M. (1988). Advocacy in nursing. *Nursing Outlook, 36*(3), 136–141.
Peters, T., & Waterman, R. (1983). *In search of excellence.* New York: Warner Books.
Research Institute of America. (1985). The nature of leadership. In *Personal report for the executive.* New York: Author.
Riddle, M. M. (1903). Address to the 6th annual convention of the Nurses' Association Alumnus of the United States. *American Journal of Nursing, 3,* 838–846.
A suggested code. (1926). *American Journal of Nursing, 26,* 599–601.
Swider, S. M., McElmurray, B. J., & Yarling, R. R. (1985). Ethical decision making in a bureaucratic context by senior nursing students. *Nursing Research, 34*(2), 108–112.
Where does loyalty end? An editorial. (1910). *American Journal of Nursing, 10,* 230–231.
Winslow, G. R. (1984). From loyalty to advocacy; a new metaphor for nursing. *The Hastings Center Report, June 14,* 32–40.
Yarling, R. R., & McElmurray, B. J. (1986). Moral foundation of nursing. *Advances in Nursing Science, Jan.,* 63–73.

2

Professional Ethics

A concern for ethical standards and a code of ethics are not unique to the profession of nursing. Other professions, within and outside of healthcare, such as medicine, law, and healthcare administration, have also formally expressed their ideals and expectations by developing a code of ethics to govern their practitioners. This endeaver proclaims to the public the commitments made by a particular professional group. As you will see in the evolution of nursing's code of ethics, nursing leaders took seriously such an undertaking. Incorporated into nursing's code are traditional concerns about what constitutes a "good" nurse, judgments based on experience, and explicit principles that ought to guide actions. The nursing code, like many others, gives a sense of history about the profession, its struggles and its triumphs. It helps guide practitioners, as new ethical issues develop. Thus position statements developed by professional organizations and groups should be able to use the Code for Nurses as a guide.

In this chapter we will first give a brief review of where professional ethics fits within the schema of ethical thinking. Then we will define such concepts as non-normative and normative ethics and differentiate the terms "morals" and "ethics." What will follow is a more intensive look at nursing's code of ethics and a comparison of it with medicine's code of ethics. Finally, we will focus on the principles that guide ethical decision making.

Where Professional Ethics Fits

Professional ethics is only one of several types of ethics. To gain a fuller appreciation for the significance of professional codes of ethics and the ethical principles that guide their tenets, we must gain a basic understanding of ethical theory. So let us begin. What is ethics? According to Beauchamp and Childress (1989), "Ethics is a generic term for several ways of examining the moral life."

Ethics is usually divided into two large divisions, non-normative ethics and normative ethics. Non-normative ethics is made up of metaethics and descriptive ethics. Metaethics is a type of ethics that philosophers use to analyze language, concepts, and thought. For example, metaethics would study the meaning of words such as "virtue", "rights," "obligation," and the like. Descriptive ethics describes what is the actual moral behavior of certain people and examines what their beliefs are as they relate to moral decision making. For example, studies performed by sociologists, anthropologists, and psychologists of the ethical behavior of various groups of people would be forms of descriptive ethics. Neither of these approaches tells us how one should act in certain situations; instead, they tell us how people actually act and reason.

The other grouping within the study of ethics, normative ethics, tells us why we ought to reason and/or act in a certain way. The study of normative ethics asks general questions such as, When is it all right to kill someone? When does doing good become harm? Normative ethics also looks at questions related to healthcare. This field of inquiry has taken on a distinct perspective within the field of ethics.

Bioethics is the study of ethics as it relates to biology and the health professions. For example, normative ethics within a bioethical context would ask if we ought to withdraw life-sustaining treatment from a patient in a persistent vegetative state, or whether we ought to give a particular patient with a history of noncompliance a second kidney transplant.

Ethics and Morals

People frequently ask what the difference is between ethics and morals, and often use the terms interchangeably. Jameton (1984) gives us an understandable way to differentiate the two words. To make the distinction clear, he contrasts the terms "professional" and "personal". The word "professional" refers to "publicly stated and formal sets of rules or values, such as professional codes of ethics". "Personal" moral values refers to more informal principles to which one is personally committed, such as "Do unto others as you would have them do unto you," "Always tell the truth," "Help those in need," and "Always keep your promise."

Some people use the term "ethics" to refer more to the systematic study of principles and values. In other words, ethics studies, questions, and inquires into what we ought to do and helps us to eventually change certain moral conduct. "Morals" refers to professional and personal convictions about how one ought to act and what one ought to believe.

Ethics thus involves a more formal approach, whereas morals is a more informal and personal term. This text will primarily focus on a formal approach to professional ethics. Yet it is difficult to separate out the informal personal moral convictions that so often guide practice. What we will do is emphasize how professional managerial practice ought to be conducted, recognizing the limits of personal and often institutional commitments.

Code for Nurses

A professional code provides guidance for carrying out the role and clarifies for society the shared professional values that guide practice. It clearly dismisses an adherence to custom and habits that do not facilitate an ethical approach to the delivery of care. "The code serves as a contract between society and the profession by explicitly setting forth the values and ethical principles that guide the clinical decisions of practicing nurses" (Murphy, 1985). The Code for Nurses provides a framework for ethical decision making and assists in identifying issues, suggesting approaches, and discriminating between alternatives.

Although all nursing professional relationships have an ethical and legal dimension, their goals and duties differ. State practice acts define standards for safe practice and set minimum standards to protect the consumer of nursing services. The Code for Nurses (Fig. 2.1), on the other hand, establishes a professional commitment and accountability that reach far beyond the law. It lets society know what it should expect from each nursing professional. The Florence Nightingale Pledge (Fig. 2.2), written by Lystra Gutter in 1893 and patterned after the Hippocratic Oath, can be considered the first code of ethics for nurses. It affirmed the nurse's commitment to confidentiality, faithfulness to patients, loyalty to physicians, and upholding standards of the profession.

The need for a professional code was recognized when nursing was first organized in 1897. The first constitution of the Nurses' Associated Alumnae Association, which was the precursor of the American Nurses' Association (ANA), cited the need to establish and maintain a professional code of ethics. It would be 50 years, however, before a

CODE FOR NURSES

1 The nurse provides services with respect for human dignity and the uniqueness of the client, unrestricted by considerations of social or economic status, personal attributes, or the nature of health problems.

2 The nurse safeguards the client's right to privacy by judiciously protecting information of a confidential nature.

3 The nurse acts to safeguard the client and the public when health care and safety are affected by the incompetent, unethical, or illegal practice of any person.

4 The nurse assumes responsibility and accountability for individual nursing judgments and actions.

5 The nurse maintains competence in nursing.

6 The nurse exercises informed judgment and uses individual competence and qualifications as criteria in seeking consultation, accepting responsibilities, and delegating nursing activities to others.

7 The nurse participates in activities that contribute to the ongoing development of the profession's body of knowledge.

8 The nurse participates in the profession's efforts to implement and improve standards of nursing.

9 The nurse participates in the profession's efforts to establish and maintain conditions of employment conducive to high quality nursing care.

10 The nurse participates in the profession's effort to protect the public from misinformation and misrepresentation and to maintain the integrity of nursing.

11 The nurse collaborates with members of the health professions and other citizens in promoting community and national efforts to meet the health needs of the public.

Figure 2.1. American Nurses' Association Code for Nurses, 1985. (Reprinted with permission from Code for Nurses with Interpretive Statements, © 1985, American Nurses' Association, Kansas City, MO.)

THE FLORENCE NIGHTINGALE PLEDGE

I solemnly pledge myself before God and in presence of this assembly:
To pass my life in purity and to practice my profession faithfully.
I will abstain from whatever is deleterious and mischievous and will not take or knowingly administer any harmful drug.
I will do all in my power to maintain and elevate the standard of my profession and will hold in confidence all personal matters committed to my keeping and family affairs coming to my knowledge in the practice of my calling.
With loyalty will I endeavor to aid the physician in his work, and devote myself to the welfare of those committed to my care.

Figure 2.2. The Florence Nightingale Pledge, 1893.

code of ethics would be adopted. Other professional priorities, such as state registration and a defined education curriculum, demanded attention. Additionally, there was disagreement about the purpose of and need for a code and confusion among nurses about what ethics is. Matters of etiquette were intermingled with ethics. Nevertheless, it preceded the publication of standards for education, practice, service, and research. Nurses in every area of practice participated in the development of a code of ethics for the profession, thus increasing its wide applicability across clinical specialties.

In 1926 the Committee on Ethical Standards of the ANA presented "A Suggested Code" to ANA convention delegates. Development of this code included input from nurses throughout the country. It highlighted the relationship of the nurse to patients, to the medical profession, to the allied professions, to other nurses, and to the nursing profession. The stated purpose was to "create a sensitiveness to ethical situations and to formulate general principles which...create the individual habit of forming conscious and critical judgment resulting in action in specific situations." This document emphasized the subservient role of the nurse, yet continually repeated that if the nurse did her job very well, she would be a co-worker with the physician. This code also emphasized strong support for nurses' involvement in professional organizations. This suggested code presented an interesting dichotomy—a dependent role with physicians and a perhaps more independent role within a larger professional context. The ANA urged the state organizations to appoint committees to study the proposed code prior to the 1928 convention. However, several years went by without much news about the suggested code.

Finally, at the 1940 ANA convention, a "tentative code" for the nursing profession was proposed by the same committee that wrote the suggested code. The first sentence of this code stated definitively that "nursing is a profession" ("A tentative code," 1940). The first section addressed the responsibility of the nurse to the profession, "reflecting the stronger identity of the nursing profession as a whole" (Vien, 1989). The tentative code had been prepared after extensive review of other professional codes and again stressed relations with the same groups as the 1926 suggested code. It also included statements about the relationship of the nurse to the employer, as well as statements about the responsibility of the nurse to herself. The section on the nurse's relationship with allied health professions now included reference to patients' families and friends (Vien, 1989).

The code clearly outlined a heritage of duty to the physician and the institution, even when personal values conflicted in carrying out physician's orders. It conceptualized the nurse as a paragon of virtue, always ready to render service, even if her own life was placed at risk. "When an epidemic prevails, she will continue her labors, with due cautions, even at risk to herself" ("A tentative code," 1940). Loyalty and obedience were also apparent virtues, taking precedence over what a nurse believed was the right thing to do.

> Because a nurse is conscientious in carrying out a physician's directions for the proper care of his patients and conforms to the rules and policies of the institution or agency in which she is serving, it need not follow that she necessarily conforms to the physician's, or others, idea of social policy. Nor does it mean that she approves of all the policies and practices of the institution or agency in which she is serving. ("A tentative code," 1940)

In 1942, when there was concern that the "tentative code" was too general to be of practical value to individual nurses, it was put into the format of a checklist and sent out for review. Copies were distributed to state associations, hospitals, nursing schools, and other healthcare professionals; 5000 were returned with comments. This input provided the basis for the first official code, which was eventually adopted at the 1950 convention. The lengthy process of developing this code, spanning the years from 1897 to 1950, seems reflective of the democratic, consensus-building processes that women typically utilize because of their socialization to work within groups, such as families. "While democratic input and consensus may result in the total group's being more committed to a decision, it is a very slow process" (Yeaworth, 1985).

Thus in 1950 the long-awaited "Code for Professional Nurses" was issued. The code stressed allegiance to the physician and the carrying out of his orders. Even though it fostered a nurse's duty to report incompetence or unethical behavior, it required such reporting to be through the appropriate administrative channels. "The nurse sustains confidence in the physician and other members of the health team; incompetency or unethical conduct of associates in the health professions should be exposed, but only to the proper authority" ("A code for nurses," 1950).

Revisions to the code occurred in 1960 and 1968. The 1960 edition delineated responsibilities for defining and upholding standards for the terms and conditions of employment and for the delegation of activities. This version deleted the ninth statement of the 1950 code, which read "The nurse has an obligation to give conscientious service and in return, is entitled to just remuneration" ("Revision proposed," 1960). That statement was eliminated because it was thought to have perpetuated a paternalistic attitude on the part of employers. Retrospectively, we must ask if its elimination has contributed to nursing's reluctance to ask for higher salaries. The 1968 version decreased the number of statements from 17 to 10 and eliminated all references to personal ethics and characteristics, changing the focus to solely that of professional behavior.

In the 1976 version of the code, 11 primary statements focused mainly on the relationship between practitioner and client, rather than the previous focus on relationships between physicians and other health professionals. It also emphasized the nurse's responsibility with regard to ethical issues in the institution, the community, and governmental decision making. It emphasized that the nurse must be responsible and accountable for individual decisions. "The nurse assumes responsibility and accountability for nursing judgments and actions"(American Nurses' Association, 1976). This code stressed the nurse's obligation to protect the patient from incompetent, illegal, or unethical medical care. It was the first time in the evolution of the code that the independent role of nursing was made clear. It was the first code to provide interpretive statements for its 11 tenets.

Major changes in the code occurred in the 1985 revision, when duty to the patient, above all else, was clearly identified. A vision of the nurse as advocate and the relationship of that role to the client's self-determination were more clearly reflected and were termed "advocacy." The 1985 version of the Code for Nurses reflects the duties, obligations, and rights of individual nurses. It gives guidance to examine and solve the current ethical issues. It exceeds the requirements in individual state practice acts. It speaks to what we ought to do, not just to what we must do. It speaks to what we are.

After almost 40 years of existence, the code has turned out to be a dynamic document, with changes occurring in it in response to changing ideas and practices and the struggles and triumphs of the nursing professions. Its basic orientation remains a concern for the dignity and welfare of the patient and for the quality and effectiveness of nursing care. The existence of a code of ethics does not automatically create an ethical profession. That requires practitioners acting as role models, actually doing what the code says each nurse ought to do. Additionally, practice environments that facilitate the code's provisions will help ensure its enforcement. "The aim of ethics is a harmonious and just society; the aim of a code is a harmonious and just profession" (Danner, 1975).

Medical Code of Ethics

The earliest written code of ethical principles for medical practice, the Code of Hammurabi, was developed in approximately 2000 B.C. by the Babylonians. This code, due to the extensive detail it contained, did not survive the test of time (Council on Ethical and Judicial Affairs of the American Medical Association [Council], 1989, p. vii). The Oath of Hippocrates, written probably sometime around 500 B.C., has been passed down through history as a brief statement of principles to guide the practice of physicians. "The Hippocratic Oath protected the rights of the patient and appealed to the inner and finer instincts of the physician without imposing sanctions or penalties on him" (Council, 1989, p. vii).

In 1803 an English physician, philosopher, and writer, Thomas Percival, published his Code of Medical Ethics. This code was used as the basis for the first Code of Ethics adopted by the American Medical Association (AMA) at their first official meeting in 1847. At that meeting, establishing a code of ethics and defining the minimum requirements for education and training were the two priorities of business. Nursing had a similar agenda at their initial organizing meeting 50 years later.

Revisions to the medical code occurred in 1903, 1912, and 1947, although the basic language and precepts remained much the same. In the mid-1950s there were attempts to reorganize the code and distinguish between matters of ethics and etiquette. This resulted in a newly formatted set of principles that was adopted by the House of Delegates at the 1957 AMA meeting. The new principles, comprised of a preamble and 10 short sections, attempted to express the fundamental concepts of the former code in a more succinct way by eliminating some ambiguous and verbose language. In 1980 major revisions were again made to clarify and update language, to eliminate reference to gender, and to provide a balance between professional guidelines and legal standards within the context of a changing society (Council, 1989, p. viii). This code now used the terminology of rights instead of a previously paternalistic notion of patient benefits: "A physician shall respect the rights of patients, of colleagues, and of other health professionals" (Council, 1989).

The current AMA Code of Ethics is comprised of three related parts: the Principles of Medical Ethics, the Current Opinions of the Council on Ethical and Judicial Affairs, and the Reports of the Council on Ethical and Judicial Affairs. The Principles include a preamble and seven precepts that define the basic standards of ethical conduct for

AMERICAN MEDICAL ASSOCIATION

PRINCIPLES OF MEDICAL ETHICS

PREAMBLE:

The medical profession has long subscribed to a body of ethical statements developed primarily for the benefits of the patient. As a member of this profession, a physician must recognize responsibility not only to patients, but also to society, to other health professionals, and to self. The following Principles adopted by the American Medical Association are not laws, but standards of conduct which define the essentials of honorable behavior for the physician.

I. **A physician shall be dedicated to providing competent medical service with compassion and respect for human dignity.**

II. **A physician shall deal honestly with patients and colleagues, and strive to expose those physicians deficient in character or competence, or who engage in fraud or deception.**

III. **A physician shall respect the law and also recognize a responsibility to seek changes in those requirements which are contrary to the best interests of the patient.**

IV. **A physician shall respect the rights of patients, of colleagues, and of other health professionals, and shall safeguard patient confidences within the constraints of the law.**

V. **A physician shall continue to study, apply and advance scientific knowledge, make relevant information available to patients, colleagues, and the public, obtain consultation, and use the talents of other health professionals when indicated.**

VI. **A physician shall, in the provision of appropriate care, except in emergencies, be free to choose whom to serve, with whom to associate, and the environment in which to provide medical services.**

VII. **A physician shall recognize a responsibility to participate in activities contributing to an improved community.**

Figure 2.3. American Medical Association's Principles of Medical Ethics, 1989. (From Council on Ethical and Judicial Affairs of the American Medical Association. *Current opinions on professional rights and responsibilities.* Chicago: American Medical Association, 1989.)

physicians (Fig. 2.3). Within the Principles, there is recognition of the physician's obligations to patients, society, the profession, and self. The Current Opinions section of the medical code provides elaboration of the principles on more than 100 specific questions related to social policy, interprofessional relations, hospital relations, advertising and media relations, fees and charges, physicians' records, practice matters, and professional rights and responsibilities. The Reports section provides detailed information on the rationale and considerations of the Council on Ethical and Judicial Affairs in reaching their opinions about ethical issues.

Comparison of Codes

When one compares elements of the Code for Nurses and the Principles of Medical Ethics, there are certainly some aspects of similarity. Both speak to providing service with respect for human dignity, the responsibility of maintaining competence by keeping current, and protecting confidentiality of patients. However, there are some notable differences that perhaps are basic to the differences between medical and nursing ethics. While the Medical Code addresses the physician's responsibility to "expose those physicians deficient in character or competence," the Code for Nurses more broadly states that "the nurse acts to safeguard the client and the public when health care and safety are affected by incompetent, unethical, or illegal practice of any person" (American Nurses Association, 1985; Council, 1989, p. ix). There is very clearly a focus on the individual physician within the medical code, while the Code for Nurses emphasizes not only the individual nurse but the profession of nursing overall. The Principles of Medical Ethics emphasizes physician's rights rather than responsibilities, such as freedom to choose their patients in nonemergency situations. The Code for Nurses focuses on the responsibilities of the nurse to individual patients and society.

Perhaps the most obvious differences are to be seen when one compares the explanatory sections that accompany each code. In the Code for Nurses, the interpretive statements go into more depth about the meaning of each item in the code itself but still remain on a broad level of definition. For example, the Code states that "the nurse assumes responsibility and accountability for individual nursing judgments and actions" (American Nurses' Association, 1985). In the interpretive statements, this is elaborated on with "accountability refers to being answerable to someone for something one has done. It means providing an explanation or rationale to oneself, to clients, to peers, to the nursing profession, and to society....Neither physicians' orders nor the employing agency's policies relieve the nurse for accountability for actions taken and judgments made" (American Nurses' Association, 1985).

When one examines the section of the medical code entitled "Current Opinions of the Council on Ethical and Judicial Affairs," which is somewhat analogous to the interpretive statements of the nursing Code, one finds something quite different. The Opinions represent a set of very narrowly defined guidelines with regard to specific issues in practice that are not necessarily directly related to one of the Principles of Medical Ethics. Some specific issues that are addressed are abortion, organ donation, relationships with nurses, advertising and publicity, fee splitting, insurance form completion charges, and sale of a medical practice (Council, 1989, p. ix).

The differences between the medical Code and the Code for Nurses are reflective perhaps of the very different way in which the two professions practice. Physicians practice in a very individualistic, isolated manner, with the primary focus being on the dyad of physician and patient. While nurses also attend to the private relationship between nurse and client, there is a far greater focus on the entire milieu or environment within which healthcare to the client is delivered, coordinated, and managed by the nurse. This difference, then, along with the inherent differences in the purposes and definitions of the two professions, perhaps explains the different focus for ethical standards and underscores the differences between nursing and medical ethics.

Ethical Principles

While the Code for Nurses provides an overall standard of ethical conduct to guide nursing practice, it does not provide specific rules, nor practical tools to direct decision making. It speaks to accepted normative principles that ought to guide choices. Likewise, a thorough understanding of the responsibilities of the nurse with regard to advocacy for the client does not necessarily assist the nurse in determining the proper thing to do within the context of a specific situation. The following section on ethical principles will provide tools to aid the nurse in decision making. Coupling these principles with the model for decision making presented in the following chapter should provide the nurse with the practical assistance necessary to sort through the dilemmas that are typically encountered in practice.

This chapter will provide a more clear understanding of the principles underlying the Code for Nurses. But before we turn to a discussion of specific principles, we now need to discuss general considerations that should be weighed when using the principles.

1. Since most situations pose ethical dilemmas in which more than one principle is applicable, complete analysis may require consideration of several principles at the same time.
2. No single ethical principle possesses sufficient weight to take precedence in all conflicting ethical claims. The strength of an individual principle depends on the uniqueness of a given situation.
3. Applying these principles allows for sound ethical judgment rather than relying on bias and intuition. Accordingly, Beauchamp and McCullough (1984) have claimed that "one must have defensible moral reasons for holding a position, and neither the position nor the reasons that underlie it can be justified if they rest solely on prejudice, emotion, false data, the authority of another individual, or claims of self-evidence (p. 11).
4. Unlike the staff nurse, the nurse manager must juggle competing obligations in an environment where management is expected to show loyalty to the organization and enhance its survival, with the latter having more and more to do with economic viability. Yet the institution has moral responsibilities to its clients. It is toward this end that the nurse manager must look when balancing competing claims on what should be done in a particular situation. Together with the model for decision making presented in Chapter 3, the principles will provide the nurse manager with the practical assistance necessary to sort through the dilemmas that are typically encountered in practice.

Bioethical Decisions

The principles we will discuss are generally applied to decision making in specific cases and have consistently raised two questions: What is the right thing to do? Who should decide? In some situations, the course of action is clear, and no one disagrees. Thus these questions do not get consciously raised. In other circumstances, the choices are not as clear. The following two cases can help illustrate this point.

A clear case: An adult patient sees his physician for abdominal pain. The pain and other symptoms lead the physician to a diagnosis of acute appendicitis. The physician explains his findings, and the patient agrees to surgery. Other healthcare providers agree with the decision. The patient has surgery, recovers in the expected time frame, and goes home. The case certainly raises the two questions mentioned above, but they do not surface because the course of action was clear, and no one disagreed. An unclear case: An adult male with amyotrophic lateral sclerosis (ALS) is placed on a ventilator. The physician believes the patient will be on the ventilator for the rest of his life. Up to this point, the patient had been at home, with increasing weakness and increasing difficulty swallowing. The physician wants to place a gastrostomy tube to deliver nutrition, and the patient has refused. In fact, this competent adult patient wants the ventilator support removed. He is very clear that he will then die. The patient has always loved his life, but does not want to live like this. His wife agrees with the decision. For others, the decision may not be so clear, and there may be disagreement. Certainly, the question about who gets to decide will be raised. In this scenario, moral issues arise that relate to futile treatment, quality of life, and patient autonomy.

The principles we will discuss mainly focus on what's the right thing to do in a specific situation. However, for the nurse, most situations raise two additional questions: What is my role? What is my responsibility? When the nurse manager asks these two additional questions, the answers she derives may be, as we shall discover, slightly different.

Autonomy

Individual freedoms are highly valued in the United States of America and are supported by our Constitution and societal norms. On the other hand, physicians and nurses in this country have traditionally approached patients paternalistically about treatment decisions. Thus patients have been denied adequate information to choose a treatment course other than that prescribed by their physician, or are entirely left out of the process by eager professionals desiring to "do good."

The ethical principle of autonomy refers to individual self-determination and freedom of choice. It requires that we respect the rights of others to make autonomous decisions. To violate a person's autonomy is to treat that person merely as a means to an end that is in accordance with one's own beliefs and values. It is difficult for health professionals to remember that the decision to accept treatment or refuse it is a moral one and not within the purview of medical decision making. "Autonomy asserts that humans have incalculable worth, deserve respect, and have the right to self determination" (Haddad, 1987).

The autonomous individual sets out a plan of action and follows through with it. Thus the patient must be informed as to the various treatment options, their risks and consequences, and the diagnosis and prognosis upon which these options are based.

Information must be provided in a language understood by the patient, with confusing medical terminology made clear. Patients must also have the time to contemplate decisions and opportunities to re-discuss their concerns. The final act of consent, or of not giving consent, must be genuinely voluntary. The ethical and legal doctrine of informed consent is based on the principle of autonomy.

Once we are sure a patient's decision is informed and freely chosen, we must respect that choice. The principle of autonomy does require us to respect a patient's choice even when we do not agree with it. "Respect involves more than taking this attitude. It involves treating agents so as to allow or to enable them to act autonomously" (Beauchamp & Childress, 1989).

Individuals unable to make decisions for themselves still have a right to have their healthcare choices honored. Patients who have completed an advance directive, indicating who is to make decisions for them and or what these decisions should be, give everyone a more clear understanding of the preferred choices. However, most patients do not complete advance directives. Surrogates, usually family members, attempt to make treatment decisions in the best interest of their loved one. Autonomous decision making can be enhanced by not waiting until competent patients become incompetent to discuss treatment options.

Certainly, there are situations when the patient's or family's refusal of treatment is believed not to be in the patient's best interest. At these times, healthcare professionals may feel compelled to "actively persuade" the patient or family to agree to treatment. It must be understood that a physician or nurse cannot possibly weigh the benefits of various treatment alternatives against an individual's own values, fears, and goals. Thus we must be clear about why we believe certain treatments should be chosen and listen carefully to the patient and or family. It must be remembered, however, that even when we believe that surrogates are not acting in the patient's best interest, we must then use the legal system for help. We cannot just do what we think is best.

Limits to Autonomy

There are limits to individual autonomy. Individuals are not free to carry out autonomous decisions that harm others. For example, physical harm, endangering the public health, disrupting another's actions, or using scarce resources indiscriminately are instances when an individual's freedom to choose a course of action may be constrained. In healthcare, the idea of a patient asking a healthcare professional to kill him using a lethal injection raises conflicts with a health professional's own values. The principle of autonomy refers to an individual's right to make decisions for himself, not others. However, American society values individual autonomy and thus requires compelling evidence to justify restricting individuals in making their own choices and directing their own lives. Autonomy is a basic right, but it is not primary in all cases.

There are instances when autonomous individuals do not want to make informed decisions. They do not want to hear all the information they might need to make a fully informed choice. A patient would thus be giving a valid consent for treatment, rather than an informed one. Documentation should reflect how the consent was obtained.

Nursing Responsibility

Physicians obtain informed consent. Nurses ensure autonomous decision making by assisting patients to understand the information provided and either carrying out their choices or making sure that no one interferes with their ability to carry out that choice. While physicians are more likely to view their role in informed consent as a single event, a study by Davis identified a broader perspective for nurses. Nurses see informed consent as a continuing process including (*a*) monitoring informed consent, (*b*) advocating for patients to the physician, (*c*) providing patients with explanations and information about alternatives, (*d*) coordinating consent processes with families and patients, and (*e*) negotiating between involved parties when there are differences of opinions (Davis, 1989).

Some individuals who may not be competent to make informed treatment decisions may be able to choose what they would like to eat or when they would like their bath. Some medical conditions, such as a transient ischemic attack (TIA) or recovery from general anesthesia, may render patients incompetent for a specific period of time. Nurses must ensure that the dependency fostered by the hospital environment, disease, or circumstance does not limit patient autonomy indefinitely. The nurse is in the best position to assess a patient's ability to make certain decisions and to ensure informedness.

Individual Nurse Autonomy

The principle of autonomy has an interesting dimension when applied to nurses themselves. Every institution, organization, or group adopts policies, procedures, and general rules of conduct. Individuals joining such a group or working within such an organization or institution are expected to follow these rules. Nurses are often asked to follow policies or implement physicians' orders with which they disagree. It is up to the nurse as an individual professional to exercise her autonomy and not blindly follow the dictates of others. The Code for Nurses states, "Nurses are accountable for judgments made and actions taken in the course of nursing practice. Neither physicians' orders nor the employing agency's policies relieve the nurse of accountability for actions taken and judgments made" (American Nurses' Association, 1985).

The Nurse Manager

Managers are obligated to respect the autonomy of individual staff members as well as patients. It is important that managers recognize an individual nurse's accountability for actions taken. A management policy that demands that nurses follow physician orders could be violating a nurse's right to not implement an order with which she disagrees. Float policies that may jeopardize patient safety and nurse competency requirements can put the nurse at significant ethical and legal risk. Policies that state a nurse must assess all patients, plan their care, and evaluate interventions are consistent with the practice of registered nurses. However, two registered nurses and 25 patients not only might make this unachievable but also flies in the face of professional obligations to clients. Nursing managers must set policies about how disputes are resolved and what nurses do in certain situations, in order to support an individual nurse's autonomy. Certainly, nursing autonomy can be curtailed by an organizational culture that strictly defines the roles and functions of the registered nurse. To recognize and impact this milieu is one of management's greatest challenges.

Beneficence and Nonmaleficence

In the area of bioethics, it is difficult to separate the principles of beneficence and nonmaleficence. Looking at these principles together, they state that

1. one ought to do or promote good,
2. one should prevent harm,
3. one should remove harmful conditions, and
4. one should not inflict harm.

The first three statements apply directly to beneficence, and the last to nonmaleficence (Beauchamp & Childress, 1989).

Beneficence is a more active principle. Whereas nonmaleficence holds that a nurse's responsibility is to do no harm, beneficence extends this obligation further by asking the nurse to actively promote good activity, remove harmful conditions, and prevent harm. Beneficence asks that we promote goods such as health, prevention of illness, and relief from pain and suffering. These concepts are consistent with what the profession believes is their responsibility. Yet when one considers doing good, certain questions must be asked: Who decides what is a good? Can circumstances alter a perception of what is good? When does doing good become doing harm? How much does an individual have to risk in order to do good?

Beneficence, Nonmaleficence, and Autonomy

Historically, in order to do good and not do harm, healthcare professionals did not inquire about patient preferences, nor share information readily. A patient's wishes, beliefs, and values were not necessarily considered relevant. Healthcare professionals wanted to protect patients from their own bad judgment and justified their actions on the basis of beneficence and nonmaleficence. Obviously, this way of thinking is in direct conflict with respect for persons.

Healthcare professionals who have difficulty discussing death and dying with families may continue to provide aggressive treatment. The family, believing there are no other viable options, are filled with guilt and conflict. The professional has indeed acted paternalistically and, in fact, may be causing much harm.

In the delivery of healthcare, there are always potential harms, even with desired interventions that promote good. It is understood that pain, discomfort, and certain side effects may occur. Nurses are obligated to institute treatment to minimize the harm, such as ensuring adequate pain medication. In the care of terminally ill patients, there is an obligation of nonmaleficence, including an obligation not to kill. There also is an obligation to beneficence, to make the patient comfortable and alleviate pain. It may be possible to alleviate pain only by hastening death. Sometimes, we fail to adequately decrease pain because of this concern and thus may actually be doing more harm. The act of alleviating pain is a good act; death is not the intended effect, nor was it necessary for the patient to die to receive relief from pain. It is important to discuss with patients and families our concerns and intended actions. We cannot assume that what we value is what others value. To ensure patient autonomy, we must allow what patients value to guide our interventions.

Benefits and Burdens

Of course, in most actions some benefits and some harms are realized. In order to apply the principles of beneficence and nonmaleficence, the benefits and burdens of treatment or nontreatment will be analyzed. Benefits such as cure, correction, or relief from pain and suffering must be weighed against the burdens identified by individuals or their surrogate decision makers. Questions such as these might be asked to help distinguish doing good from doing harm:

- What is the degree of intrusiveness, risk, and discomfort of treatment?
- Will the intervention minimize or relieve pain?
- Does the treatment prolong an inevitable death?
- Can the patient's prognosis be improved?
- What is the individual's capacity to experience and enjoy life?
- What are the possibilities of a return to cognitive life and a physically functioning life?

Should we take into account the social as well as the physical burdens generated by a potential treatment? For example, should we give a heart transplant to a patient known for his poor eating and drinking habits? Should we pursue aggressive treatment for premature infants under 700 grams when the family cannot bear the cost of care? Should we continue to treat an infant with debilitating chronic disease when we know that the baby lives amidst poverty and emotional deprivation? Some of these situations and others like them make us question what we are doing. Yet, social conditions are not morally relevant criteria by which to deny treatment. Certainly, a policy that allowed us to consider socially induced burdens would most likely impede any efforts to improve the situation and be a setup for moral discrimination.

One of the most difficult situations in which to weigh benefits and burdens is when there is medical uncertainty, when the precise diagnosis and/or prognosis is unclear. Sometimes further tests, consultations, and/or family conferences will clarify facts, minimize assumptions, and facilitate decision making. Sometimes the passage of time makes clear the likely extent of recovery. In these and other situations, "moral uncertainty" (Jameton, 1984) may persist because it is not known which courses of action are permitted, obligated, and/or prohibited. For example, in the past, it was believed that a physician needed more justification to stop treatment than to actually not begin it at all. Court cases and ethical guidelines have proven that premise false. Once treatment is started, there is not a commitment to continue it. Sometimes therapy is initiated or patients are resuscitated because time is needed to make a decision. All the facts may not be known and/or the patient and family has not had a chance to discuss alternatives. All too often, healthcare professionals do not stop and ask if what they are doing is good for the patient. They allow the patient's interests to get buried under sophisticated medical procedures and technically demanding management decisions.

Due Care

Nurses must practice with due care to ensure minimal and avoidable harm. To be morally blameworthy, a harm must be caused by a failure to comply with a social, legal, or moral duty. What constitutes that duty is impacted by state practice acts, laws, regulations, and current acceptable standards of practice. A nurse is held to a community standard for practice, whether it is adhered to at her particular institution or not. A nurse manager who is not open to new ways of doing things and does not ensure that current clinical concepts are part of policies and procedures may prevent a nurse from exercising due care. Tenet 5 of the Code for Nurses states, "The nurse maintains competence in nursing" (American Nurses' Association, 1985). Practicing with due care requires sufficient knowledge, skill, and ability to recognize when more information is needed. Failing to position a patient appropriately in bed or on the operating table can lead to avoidable harms such as contractures, foot-drop, bruising, or decreased motion. Were these outcomes to have occurred, the nurse would not have practiced with due care.

The Role of Nursing Management

It is up to nursing management to minimize institutional barriers that interfere with the nurse's ability to practice safely and within expected standards of care. The nurse manager must ensure the presence of needed and functioning equipment, necessary supplies, adequate staffing, and current policies and procedures. Thus the staff nurse should be able to practice safely and minimize harm.

The nurse manager also has affirmed loyalty to the institution. Her job is to enforce the policies, procedures, and rules that may often be set by others. Yet the nurse manager also has obligations to patients. Take for example this situation: There is a nursing department policy that all nurses must float from unit to unit to meet staffing needs. There is no limitations as to where a nurse might be expected to practice on a given day. The policy further states that part-time nurses float before full-time nurses. Today, the nurse manager of the postpartum area must float a nurse to the infectious disease unit. The only part-time nurse on duty has worked postpartum only for the last 10 years. The nurse manager has some choices. She could simply enforce the policy, and the staff nurse could comply. The nurse manager could enforce the policy, and the staff nurse could refuse to float, based on her concerns about her knowledge base. Seeing these alternatives as the only two options limits a nurse manager's ability to ensure a safe environment for staff and patients. Thus the nurse manager could consider other options before making a choice. The nurse manager could override the policy and float a full-time nurse. The nurse manager could float the part-time nurse and help ensure that the assignment would not put the nurse or patients at risk. The nurse manager could review staffing in the entire hospital and designate another unit where the nurse could float. The nurse manager's obligation is to weigh the likely consequences of each option and chose the one that will result in the most good for patients and staff and not inflict harm for all concerned in the situation.

Justice

The concept of justice is discussed more fully in the chapter on allocation of nursing resources.

Fidelity

Fidelity refers to faithfulness or promise keeping. Beauchamp and Childress (1989) believe fidelity to be a rule derived from the four principles described above. Ramsey (1970) argues that fidelity is actually the foundational principle from which other principles arise. Certainly fidelity, as it relates to commitment, is basic to the relationship nurses establish with patients. Promises to provide and meet a patient's care needs are implicit in the obligations nurses make to society.

Promises may be implicit or explicit. The implicit promise is related to the fundamental relationship of the nursing profession to society. There is dependence on the nurse not to abandon patients and to look after their needs, as well as to advocate for patients in situations where they are unable to represent their own interests adequately. Explicit promises may also be made by a nurse to a specific patient, for example, making a promise to minimize pain or teach home care. Sometimes these promises are difficult to keep, due to other circumstances or conflicting obligations. Fidelity relates to the keeping of promises; thus inherent in this concept is the necessity that the nurse give careful consideration before making promises.

Veracity

Obligations of veracity are derived from obligations of fidelity, autonomy, beneficence, and nonmaleficence. Veracity requires that we tell the truth and not intentionally deceive or mislead others. Deception can occur in three ways:

1. By not disclosing information
2. By disclosing only partial information
3. By lying

In healthcare, it has been common practice not to tell the truth when we believe it may harm the patient. Beauchamp and Childress (1989) note that medical codes of ethics have generally ignored the rule of veracity. However, the 1980 revision of the Principles of Medical Ethics states that the physician should "deal honestly with patients and colleagues" (Council, 1989). The Code for Nurses states the position of the nursing profession more emphatically: "Truth telling and the process of reaching informed choice underlie the exercise of self-determination, which is basic to respect for persons" (American Nurses' Association, 1985).

At the core of the relationship between nurse and patient is a recognition that truth telling will occur. Lying, which threatens that relationship, fails to show respect for persons and threatens the nurse-patient relationship. The burden of proof must be on the healthcare professional to show that deception is the only way to do good. In fact, the nurse must look to other alternatives instead of actively lying to a patient, even if they involve additional time, energy, or money, to ensure truth telling. For example, a nurse who knows that a patient is being denied sufficient information about her prognosis must contact the physician and, failing this, should see out other resources to ensure patient informedness. Consider this situation: A patient had been asking the nurse to contact her physician. The patient had some additional questions about the surgery that was scheduled in the morning. The nurse said she would do what was asked and, in fact, followed through on repeated occasions. The nurse left a message at the physician's office to call the nursing unit, stating Mrs. Wright's concerns. Three hours later the nurse paged the physician, who failed to respond. Approximately 2 hours later the physician arrived on the nursing unit, read his patient's chart, wrote some orders, and was about to leave the unit when he was stopped by the nurse. The nurse asked the physician if he got her message. The physician stated that he had but was too busy to deal with Mrs. Wright. He told the nurse to tell Mrs. Wright that he was unavailable till morning. Certainly, the nurse has an obligation not to lie to the patient. In fact, the nurse has a further obligation to let the physician know that she will not follow his instructions and will tell the patient that he was here, was spoken to by the nurse, but did not wish to see the patient at this time. Any other response would tempt the nurse to fashion a "white lie" in order to do what the physician asks, by saying something like this: "Mrs. Wright, I just saw your physician, but he is on his way to an emergency and will see you as soon as he can." This type of lying has been called benevolent deception and is not morally justifiable. It does not show respect for persons, nor does it take into account the long-term consequences of lying. Continuing this pattern of deception would ultimately destroy the trust the patient has in the nurse.

The Nurse Manager

The nurse manager, as a representative of the institution, has made promises to patients and the institution. The hospital represents a safe, trustworthy environment. Patients trust that the management ensures an environment free of obvious hazards, with safe equipment, adequate supplies, and competent staff. Obviously, iatrogenic complications can arise that may be due to a failure of equipment or an incompetent staff member. A nurse manager owes the patient truthfulness about the cause of the problem and information on how the problem will be corrected. One of the pitfalls, particularly in situations involving a nurse, is when the patient insists that the nurse be disciplined and/or terminated. The patient does have the right to the truth, and to be assured that this occurrence will be prevented in the future, but does not have the right to know the sanctions, if any, that were taken against the nurse. Disciplinary action is between the nurse and the manager and divulging the specific disciplinary action to the patient would deny the nurse's own right to privacy. The patient would have to pursue legal action to achieve any other desired end. The nurse manager's obligation to the institution would be met if (*a*) a thorough investigation was conducted, (*b*) appropriate verbal and/or written feedback was given to the patient, (*c*) the appropriate hospital representatives (such as the chief nursing officer, the hospital administrator, and the risk manager) were informed, (*d*) the nurse was treated fairly by receiving discipline consistent with the findings and in a way others in similar circumstances would be treated.

The Concept of Risk

In order to do good and not do harm, sometimes in order to keep promises or tell patients the truth, a nurse will have to take a risk. Must the nurse act, even in the face of significant personal risk? Can the nurse manager expect a nurse to act in these situations?

Some nurses work with patients with unknown diseases or patients receiving experimental drugs. Nurses accept this risk as part of their practice. A nurse manager who hires a nurse, explaining the types of patients to be cared for, can expect the nurse to do so. However, even under these conditions, a nurse manager could not expect the nurse to care for some of the patients on the unit without adequate protection. For example, when caring for certain patients with communicable respiratory disease, masks and cover gowns should be available. In this era of universal precautions, a nurse should not be expected to draw blood or handle any body secretions without the availability of gloves and goggles.

Smith and Davis (1980) divide the concept of risk into low, moderate, and high. Low risk involves clinical situations where no known protections are necessary when giving care, and when institutional policies and rules do not put the nurse in a precarious ethical and or legal position. Moderate risk exists when there is potential harm for the nurse. With the appropriate protection, the above-mentioned clinical situations would be considered moderate risks, and the nurse would be obligated to give care. A moderate risk for the nurse might occur when policies support a nurse's questioning of physician orders, but the institutional norm is that with certain physicians, this just does not occur.

High-risk situations would pose considerable personal risk for the nurse, for example, entering a burning room to save a patient and caring for patients with known communicable diseases for which there is no assured protection. Nurses who are pregnant would be putting their unborn children at high risk if they had to care for a child with active rubella disease. Management must assure that nurses are not obligated to render care in these high-risk situations. The chapter on whistleblowing will identify some of the high-risk situations that a nurse could find herself in, when protecting unsafe or incompetent practice.

Summary

The Florence Nightingale Pledge includes the promise "I will abstain from whatever is deleterious and mischievous, . . . and devote myself to the welfare of those committed to my care." The ANA's Code for Nurses (1985) has language that is similar: "The nurse's primary commitment is to the health, welfare, and safety of the client." However, it is obvious that implementation of these high standards is not so simple. The duty to benefit the client may come into direct conflict with other ethical duties, such as not doing harm, respecting the autonomy of patients, or allocating scarce resources. Awareness that these concepts are interwoven will help the nurse be more accountable for actions done on behalf of patients. An understanding of the concepts that ought to guide professional practice will help the manager grapple with the ethical issues that arise in today's healthcare institutions.

REFERENCES

American Nurses' Association. (1976). *Code for nurses with interpretive statements.*Kansas City, MO: Author.

American Nurses' Association. (1985). *Code for nurses with interpretive statements.* Kansas City, MO: Author.

Beauchamp, T. L., & Childress, J. F. (1989). *Principles of biomedical ethics* (3rd ed.). New York: Oxford University Press.

Beauchamp, T. L. & McCullough, L. B. (1984). *Medical ethics: The moral responsibilities of physicians.* Englewood Cliffs, NJ: Prentice-Hall.

A code for nurses. (1950). *American Journal of Nursing, 50,* 196.

Council on Ethical and Judicial Affairs of the American Medical Association. (1989). *Current opinions on professional rights and responsibilities.* Chicago: Author.

Danner, C. K. (1975). Medical ethics: Some uses, abuses, and limitations. *New England Journal of Medicine, 293,* 384–387.

Davis, A. J. (1989). Clinical nurses' ethical decision making in situations of informed consent. *Advances in Nursing Science, 12,* 63–69.

Haddad, A. (1987). Ethics: Using principles of beneficence and autonomy to resolve ethical dilemmas in perioperative nursing. *Association of Operating Room Nurses Journal, 46,* 120–124.

Jameton, J. (1984). *Nursing practice—the ethical issues.* Englewood Cliffs, NJ: Prentice-Hall.

Murphy, C. P. (1985). *Ethical dilemmas in nursing practice.* Kansas City, MO: American Nurses' Association.

Ramsey, P. (1970). *The patient as person.* New Haven, CT: Yale University Press.

Revision proposed in code for professional nurses. (1960). *American Journal of Nursing, 60,* 80–81.

Smith, S. J., & Davis, A. J. (1980). Ethical dilemmas: Conflicts among rights, duties, and obligations. *American Journal of Nursing, 80,* 1463–1466.

A suggested code. (1926). *American Journal of Nursing, 26,* 599–601.

A tentative code for the nursing profession. (1940). *American Journal of Nursing, 40,*977–980.

Vien, D. C. (1989). A history of nursing's code of ethics. *Nursing Outlook, 37*(1), 45–49.

Yeaworth, R. C. (1985). The ANA code: A comparative perspective. *Image: The Journal of Nursing Scholarship, 17*(3), 94–98.

3

Ethical Decision Making

Advances in scientific knowledge and technologic applications have caused healthcare professionals to take a more critical look at the ethical aspects of the care they deliver. In an era of an increasing aged population, decreasing healthcare reimbursement, and increasing consumer demand for autonomous decision making, ethical issues are being pushed into the limelight. In the past, the issues seemed less complicated and fewer in number. Caring, compassion, and a desire to do the right thing were all one needed. Today, new and difficult questions make many decisions appear impossible. The issues can be life threatening and thus emotionally charged, necessitating rapid, assertive intervention. One study demonstrated that one out of every six cases on a general medical ward of a university hospital presented serious ethical problems. It also pointed out that sensitization to ethical concerns and an informed, sympathetic listener increased awareness of ethical problems (Lo & Schraeder, 1981).

Ethical decision making is a complex process. It is based on sorting out what is the right thing to do amidst personal, professional, and societal values. The process recognizes that individuals' knowledge about ethical principles and their level of moral reasoning influence choices. Ketefian (1981) and Langham (1977) have shown that the cognitive processes nurses use in making decisions about moral issues are mostly individualistic, intuitive, and commonsense processes rather than well-reasoned and well-informed ones. Thus many nurses tend to choose the "easiest" decision path, going on with their work and then sharing their feelings at shift report or over lunch, or thinking about it in their dreams. The general lack of ethics content in nursing education and the subsequent socialization process do not reward independent thinking or creative activities. Instead, obedience, courtesy, and competent task performance are valued. As Yarling and McElmurray (1986) point out, students are verbally taught one way to act, and nonverbally another. In another study by Swider, McElmurray, and Yarling (1985) of ethical decision making by senior nursing students, three categories of nursing responses were used to classify the decisions students made. The categories were patient centered, physician centered, and bureaucratic centered. A majority of the responses were bureaucratic centered, as the students typically sought first to abide by rules within the system. The study also pointed out the students' general confusion about a nurse's ultimate responsibility in sorting out ethical issues.

Kohlberg's (1976) theory of moral development helps us understand why two intelligent, committed nurses may arrive at different ethical decisions in the same situation. Kohlberg's theory identifies three levels of moral development, with two stages in each level. At the first level, preconventional, the individual is self-centered and narcissistic. In stage 1 of this level, the individual defines what is right and wrong according to what will win him rewards or punishment. In stage 2, the individual reciprocates to get the result he wants.

The second level is called conventional and is society focused. What is right and what is wrong are determined from external sources. Here, in the third stage, parents, priests, and teachers (in other words, authority figures) are looked to for guidance. In the fourth stage, the focus moves from personal to impersonal authority, such as laws, religious precepts, and so on.

The third level is called postconventional and is humanity centered. Self-chosen ethical principles supercede the demands of laws. In the fifth stage, individuals determine the rightness or wrongness of an act by its ability to achieve the greatest good for the greatest number. Individuals reaching the sixth stage look to the concept of justice to aid in their decision making.

Take the situation where a decision must be made about withholding or withdrawing life support on a particular patient. One nurse may be operating at stage 4 in her moral development and depend on written policies and laws for guidance. A nurse responding from stage 5 would be more likely to evaluate how the patient's suffering is impacting him and his family.

The significance of this theory lies in its explanation of the relationships between moral reasoning and moral action. At higher stages of moral reasoning, there is a greater likelihood that one will resist the pressure of compromising oneself and thus tend to act morally. However, it is important to recognize that Kohlberg's stages reflect how one reasons about one's moral choices, not necessarily how one acts. Understanding what one values goes hand in hand with this concept. "Values are general guides to behaviors, standards of conduct that one endorses and uses to live up to" (Ustal, 1978). The clearer nurses are about what they value, the more they are able to choose a course of action that maintains their integrity. The result will be more independent moral judgments and less conformity with others' beliefs. This position has also been supported by Yarling and McElmurray (1986). It also must be stated that making a decision based on one's values implies an understanding of the consequences of the decision and its impact on others.

It is not the intent of this book to explore the relationship in depth, but nursing managers must recognize the significance of a nurse's moral development and the subsequent implications that has for her role within the institution. When discussing ethical issues, even in the best of situations, "ethical choices remain hard choices . . . because they make conflicting claims on us, or present us with seemingly equally unsatisfactory choices" (Smith & Davis, 1980).

Interestingly and unfortunately, in spite of an individual nurse's own moral development, many writers have concluded that nurses in general suffer fundamental moral dilemmas because of their role as nurses. Mitchell (1981) emphasized that nurses confront ethical dilemmas when mutually exclusive expectations are placed on them. For example, the patient expects the nurse to be honest and caring, the physician expects the nurse to be obedient, and nursing management expects the nurse to follow the rules and not make waves. Studies by Grey-Toft and Anderson (1981), Jacobson (1987), and Oskins (1979) reported that for nurses, the most stressful aspect of the job centered around moral and ethical problems. Curtain (1980) stated that "the major ethical dilemma in nursing is that nurses are not free to practice nursing." She believes that the nurse is constantly constrained by a bureaucratic, paternalistic environment.

Anatomy of a Dilemma

An ethical dilemma may occur when there is a conflict among duties, loyalties, rights, and/or values. Clinically, the issues have to do with determining the morally right thing to do in a given patient care situation and/or with determining who decides a certain treatment direction. If everyone is in agreement about the choice to be made, there is no dilemma. Sometimes, though, questions arise as to the benefits or harms related to certain choices, or whether specific individuals have the "right" to make certain decisions that others may not perceive to be correct. When there is disagreement among the members of the healthcare team and/or with the patient and family, an ethical dilemma may be created.

Likewise, management issues arise that may have moral considerations but not necessarily pose an ethical dilemma, unless there is disagreement about the right thing to do or who should decide. For example, a nurse manager believes that the budgeted hours per patient day (HPPD) for her unit are insufficient for patient acuity. If the budget is augmented once brought to administration's attention, the issue is resolved, and a potential moral conflict is avoided. However, if the manager is told that there can be no additional hours budgeted, regardless of patient acuity, the nurse manager is faced with an ethical dilemma. How can safe care be delivered to patients? Will harm occur? Certainly, in this situation, the manager's role obligations are in direct conflict with her duty to do good and not harm the patients.

In a dilemma, the choices usually appear to be equally unsatisfactory, not readily evident, or in need of delineation. Smith and Davis (1980) suggest that an ethical dilemma arises in the following situations:

1. There is a conflict between two equally unsatisfactory alternatives. An example of this might be the situation where there is no nurse for the oncoming shift to staff the labor and delivery area. What choices does the nurse manager have? To float a medical surgical nurse in to staff labor and delivery or leave the area unstaffed and refuse admissions. Neither choice is satisfactory. Each has consequences that compromise patient safety.
2. There is a conflict between two ethical principles one holds. The example above could hold true here as well. The two ethical principles in conflict are beneficence and nonmaleficence, the choice between doing good and doing harm. With either choice the manager could end up doing harm in an attempt to do good, and patient safety could be jeopardized.
3. There is a conflict between one's ethical principles and one's role obligations. An operating room nurse is required by the institution to care for all assigned patients. A physician is going to perform a second kidney transplant on a very elderly, frail patient. The nurse does not support this decision and wonders what the patient was told about the risks. The nurse is also wondering about the physician's decision to use a scarce resource (the donated organ) on this

particular patient. The nurse could refuse to care for this patient. The risk in some institutions could be disciplinary action or the possible loss of her job for refusing an assignment. But if she cares for the patient, she may be compromising the principles she values.

4. There is a demand for action and a need for reflection. One example of this could be when a terminally ill patient arrests, but there is no Do Not Resuscitate order. What should be done? There is a demand for action, but a need for reflection.

A Model for Decision Making

A model to aid in decision making is described below (Fig. 3.1). The purpose of ethical discussion is to subject dilemmas to systematic, rational analysis. Such analysis includes the collection of accurate information, application of appropriate ethical principles, the exploration of all reasonable options and their consequences, and the selection of a course of action. A systematic approach to analyzing these dilemmas will help the practitioner grapple more easily with the issues, clarify thoughts, and bring illumination to difficult choices. This process should decrease the influence of misinformation, individual bias, and incomplete consideration, and thus result in a better decision. Yet

I. Define the dilemma.

II. Identify the medical facts.

III. Identify the nonmedical facts.
   A. Patient and family.
   B. External influences.

IV. Separate assumptions from facts.

V. Identify items needing clarification.

VI. Identify the decision makers.

VII. Review underlying ethical principles.

VIII. Define alternatives.

IX. Follow-up.

Figure 3.1. A model for ethical decision making. (© Levine-Ariff, J. & Groh, D. 1987. Reprinted with permission.)

> coming to the 'right' answer ethically does not necessarily free us from the personal pain of a situation: it simply clarifies the moral appropriateness of an alternative, provides us with greater confidence, and frees us from vague but gnawing feelings of guilt, apprehension or doubt. (Fowler, 1987)

At first glance, the model may appear cumbersome and unwieldy. It is important to reflect back to learning the scientific method and the nursing process. Remember how these steps shed light on approaches to problems, which now require little conscious thought. Ethical issues require a different method of analysis, a new approach for different types of decisions. When used, this model too will become second nature and an integral part of daily practice. When using the model for cases that are not clinical in nature, such as staffing or impaired professionals, some steps of the model may be less relevant. The examples at the end of the chapter should make the differences clear.

When analyzing an ethical dilemma, the clinical aspects of the case become the backdrop for an organized discussion of the dilemma and possible solutions. A clinical dilemma can often be discussed in a group setting, while a management issue that presents a dilemma may frequently be processed by a single individual or one-to-one with another individual.

The Steps of the Model

I. Define the Dilemma

The first step in any problem-solving method is to define the issue. Since ethical dilemmas are sometimes difficult to state succinctly, just state the concern in your own words. For example, "Dr. Johnson is not telling Mrs. Stone the truth about her prognosis," or "I don't think Mr. Stevens wants his wife on the ventilator any longer, but Dr. Marks won't discuss this with him." In a group, verbalize the thoughts of all the members so a consensus can be reached on the problem(s). Members may have different agendas, and the discussion could ramble, with individuals focusing on personal thoughts and personal preferences.

Sometimes the identified dilemma will not be an ethical one but an administrative or communication problem. It is important to recognize this as soon as possible and proceed with other appropriate problem-solving approaches, rather than continuing with this model. For example, in one situation where a nurse and resident called for a consultation by the Institutional Ethics Committee (IEC), they believed there existed a conflict between what the patient and family wanted (nontreatment) and what the attending physician wanted (treatment). In the discussion that ensued, the attending agreed that the patient's life was nearing an end and no treatment would cure or even restore any function. The attending said he did not realize how strongly the patient and family felt about wanting to go home and letting life or death take its natural course. The conference ended with a plan to see the family immediately and facilitate discharge. In this situation, there was no dilemma because everyone agreed on the decision to be made. The problem had been one of poor or inadequate communication between the various individuals involved.

Likewise, it is important to avoid confusing legal questions with ethical dilemmas. Certainly, a clarification of the legal position may be necessary, but it is important to remember that moral decision making may or may not be supported by law. For example, practitioners often ask the question, "Can we legally withdraw support on this patient?" before they have fully discussed the matter. Is it or is it not in this patient's best interests to have life support withdrawn? What are the patient's preferences? What does the family want to do? These questions must be asked and answered first. Then, look to the legal questions.

II. Identify the Medical Facts

In delineation of the medical facts, it may become apparent that some individuals see the facts differently from others. Facts that were thought to be accurate may not be. The consequences of various medical interventions must be clear, as well as the expected benefits to the patient. Conflicts between different medical specialists need to be acknowledged and explored. Diagnosis and prognosis should be confirmed and understood by all, or discrepancies raised.

Critical in this discussion is the issue of relevancy. Too often, when learning ethical decision making, nurses and physicians get bogged down in the medical model and spend a great deal of time discussing the intricacies of various medical tests, treatments, and responses. It is tempting to pursue analysis of the electrolyte results or the latest hemogram because these are tangibles that we understand and can usually manipulate to our satisfaction. Discussions can easily go off on tangents about the latest experimental interventions or research findings that would probably not have been considered, were it not for the issue at hand. This is not to say that such discussion should be cut off, but it is important when discussing the ethical concerns to keep everyone focused on the relevancy of such issues to the dilemma at hand.

Managerial issues that lead to ethical questions may also present situations where the medical "facts" need to be clarified. Assumptions about certain types of behavior may lead a manager to inappropriately "label" an employee and apply disciplinary action that may not be justified. Using terms such as "neurotic," "psychotic," or "alcoholic" instead of objective descriptions of behavior such as "short attention span," "slurred speech," or "lapses in memory" may obscure a serious medical problem and severely compromise a manager's ability to treat people fairly. It is very important that this information be clear, objective, and factual. No matter whether the behavior is caused by a medical problem, substance abuse, or psychiatric illness, the manager's responsibility is to ensure that no harm comes to patients and that the employee is treated with compassion and respect and offered appropriate help.

III. Identify the Nonmedical Facts

There are two distinct groups of nonmedical facts: those that apply directly to the patient and family and those that are external, yet may indirectly or directly affect them and/or the alternatives that may be identified to resolve the dilemma.

Patient and Family

Family demographics, cultural factors, religious beliefs, and the social and psychological history of the patient and family can be important information and should be identified at this point. The existence of living wills, durable powers of attorney for health care, or verbal statements made by patients indicating values or preferences in such situations should also be discussed. How a person lived his or her life can also be an important piece of data to aid in determining preferences for the incompetent patient. What the patient and family "know" about the issue at hand should be openly discussed. Sometimes what some health care providers believe the family knows is not always based on fact. Relevancy is a key factor here as well. It is very easy to get caught in the intricacies of the psychosocial data. The statement of the dilemma should periodically be reinforced so that relevancy is maintained and gossip is minimized.

External Influences

Administrative policies, federal and state laws, practice acts, regulations, professional codes of ethics, and nursing and medical standards of care should be considered, as applicable to the situation. This is where the values of the healthcare providers should be identified, and any conflict with the patient's family's value system acknowledged. It is imperative that we do not attempt to answer ethical dilemmas by asking the question, "What would you do if it were you, your mother, father, or child?" The fact is that this is not you or your mother, father, or child under discussion and that question could be answered by three different people in three different ways. What we can be reasonably sure of is that each individual would probably want the autonomy to make decisions about his/her own or his/her family member's care.

When stating facts of policies, procedures, laws, and regulations in the course of an ethical discussion, one must recognize that ethics asks what "ought to be" and weighs current practices in that light. Perhaps the situation under consideration will alter a now-current institutional practice. The law can be a tool or a barrier, and what is legal is not always ethical. Establishing the legality of an action does not speak to its morality, yet known laws or legal precedents should be acknowledged and discussed. Certainly, if a state or federal law clearly forbids a certain action to take place, legal counsel should be sought, and risks and consequences identified. Current healthcare practices are presenting new ethical issues that will often be ahead of changes in the law and institutional policies. This is perhaps a mixed blessing. While offering no constraints, there is also no guidance imposed by others who have discussed the issue and made decisions. We must remember that the law requires us to do no harm, while ethics requires us to also do good.

IV. Separate Assumptions from Facts

As the medical and nonmedical facts are identified, it becomes clear that certain facts are really just assumptions. Too often we misinterpret an individual's statement. We must listen carefully and ensure separation of fact and assumption. An example would be if we interpret a family's statement of "We don't want him to suffer" as meaning they want life support withdrawn or no resuscitation, when really their concern is focused on ensuring adequate pain relief. Frequently, by virtue of an individual's stated religion, an assumption is made that he/she would make certain choices, when indeed he/she may have entirely different preferences. In management issues, for example, it may be easy for a nurse manager to be swayed by a physician's allegations that a nurse was negligent in her care of his patients, particularly when authoritarian and articulate language convey the concern. However, the facts must be clearly separated from assumptions. In this situation, it is up to the nurse manager to gather relevant and accurate information.

V. Identify Items That Need Clarification

It is often the assumptions that fall into the area of needing clarification. In addition, other information needed will usually be identified as part of the process in steps II and III.

VI. Identify the Decision Makers

The identification of the decision maker is an important step toward fitting the pieces of the puzzle together. Is the patient an adult, competent to make healthcare choices? If not, has a surrogate decision maker been identified, and by whom? Have the preferences of the child patient been taken into account? Children from the age of 7 are felt to be capable of stating preferences on how they would like to be treated. Certainly, adolescents have reached the age of assent. Although unable to give legal consent for treatment, their preferences must be weighed heavily. Many states have laws that define certain situations when a minor can grant legal permission for treatment. Be sure to review state or hospital association consent manuals that contain this information, or consult legal counsel.

Too often, the decision maker is automatically considered to be the physician. A nursing dilemma places the nurse in a position as the decision maker. It must also be remembered that while many dilemmas place the physician and nurse in positions of concern and advisory capacity to the patient, it is the patient, or the family as the surrogate decision maker, who actually decides the course of treatment. It is helpful to distinguish between medical decisions and those decisions that are moral in nature. Decisions that require medical diagnosis, prognosis, and proposed treatment are ones in which physicians have specific expertise. Decisions about whether or not to proceed with recommended treatments are moral ones that must be made by the patient/family based on their values. We must be careful not to give power to individuals for decisions that are not theirs to make.

VII. Review Underlying Ethical Principles

Principles of bioethics can be employed as guides for making moral decisions and as standards for the evaluation of actions and policies. They help us recognize what is really happening. If we say a patient has just had a stroke, certain images form in our mind. We begin to formulate questions and, based on the answers, prepare for certain interventions. In the same way, if we identify an issue as one of patient autonomy, certain questions will surface, and potential direction to resolve the issue will emerge. The ethical principles that are pertinent to a given dilemma need to be discussed. A discussion of ethical principles that can be used to guide decision making can be found in Chapter 2.

Most dilemmas do not have just one principle operating. Discussion may clarify one principle as currently being the most important. It may become evident during the discussion that various members of the group hold certain principles as more important than others. For example, for certain practitioners, doing no harm may be more important than doing good. Understanding the ethical principles helps us to separate out the healthcare professional's values from the patient's or family's values. Clarification of this will aid in the delineation of alternatives and make choices more clear.

VIII. Define Alternatives

At this point, only one alternative may be identified as the natural and obvious choice. However, discussion may identify multiple alternatives. To determine appropriate actions, one needs to weigh the options generated against the principles and/or values involved. Value considerations for the nurse manager may be to act fairly, to be an advocate for her staff, to ensure that staff are performing at a particular level of competency, and so forth. Discussion is important. Sometimes this leads to clearer thinking on why a certain alternative is predominating. It further clarifies why a particular decision is made, and not another.

It is important not to immediately squelch those alternatives that seem unacceptable. It may be that some alternatives are unacceptable only on the surface or only to some of the group. The reality might be that what seems to be an unacceptable alternative initially is really quite viable, except for institutional barriers such as arbitrary or outdated policies. It may be that these barriers need to be eliminated or minimized, and the process to do so may be listed as an alternative. Those options that are truly identified as unacceptable need to be raised and then dismissed. Acknowledgment of unacceptable alternatives is just as important as acknowledgment of reasonable ones. It may help the healthcare team to understand the issue more fully.

Some alternatives to ethical issues do not have the luxury of time. A staff nurse tells the nurse manager about finding a physician in a patient's room doing repeated lumbar punctures without additional pain medication. Against the protests of the nurse, the physician proceeded with the procedure. When the nurse refused to assist in the procedure, the physician got the medical student to hold the patient still. Although the actual situation is no longer occurring at this moment, the nurse manager has two obligations in this situation. She has an immediate obligation to ensure that this patient and other patients do not suffer preventable harm (pain). The nurse manager also needs to clarify with the staff nurse what her duty was. Protecting the patient from harm may mean "interfering" with a procedure and not allowing the physician to continue. The nurse manager needs to provide guidance on how one could do this and then discuss with the nurse how to tell the physician he was causing avoidable harm to this patient and that she (the nurse) would not allow him to proceed with the procedure. The nurse manager then should explain to the staff nurse how she plans to pursue this issue through the hospital and medical staff organizational channels, to prevent future occurrences.

IX. Follow-Up

Once the acceptable alternatives have been identified, it is important to designate the process that will be followed to reach resolution of the dilemma. It is here that, in a group process, individuals will be designated to obtain additional information and/or validate certain facts, as identified under section V. The alternatives could be prioritized, or a clear decision path defined. It may be necessary to reconvene the group once that information is obtained to decide final resolution. Or, the nurse presenting the dilemma may be the only one to follow through with a particular alternative. To whom and how the discussion conclusions will be communicated needs to to be defined. Additionally, thought should be given to whether education may be needed. Also, are policies or guidelines needed to address similar situations in the future? Has this issue arisen before? A nurse manager can be particularly helpful at this point, depending upon the alternatives chosen. Institutional policies may need to be clarified, and resources may need to be identified. The nurse manager's position in the organization and her ability to access information from various hierarchial levels can facilitate a more positive and rapid outcome.

Once the alternatives have been implemented, it is important to reconvene the individuals involved in the decision making. If the outcome was satisfactory and the process was a reasonable one, the participants need that recognition. However, if the outcome and/or the process was less than desirable, it is helpful to discuss what could be done differently next time. This type of follow-up also allows for feelings of dissatisfaction to surface and for recognition that sometimes, even when the "right" thing is done, moral tragedy still results. Providing opportunities for expression of these feelings helps relieve the internal moral stress that often accompanies ethical decision making.

Recommended Uses for the Model

The ethical decision making model can be viewed as a problem-solving methodology. However, not all dilemmas need to be, or should be, subjected to group process. It may be one individual nurse, two nurses, or a nurse with another individual who discusses the issues.

When immediate decisions are required, it may be impossible to spend the time this model necessitates. However, as one works with the model in both prospective and retrospective case review, it will serve as an aid for quickly processing the known and the unknown pieces of information and arriving at alternatives for action. As one gains confidence with the model and with ethical discussion, some steps may require only brief consideration and need not be followed in a rigid sequence. Figure 3.2 shows how the various steps of the model are interrelated and do not necessarily need to be followed sequentially. Decision making is a process, not an act. Procedural knowledge is

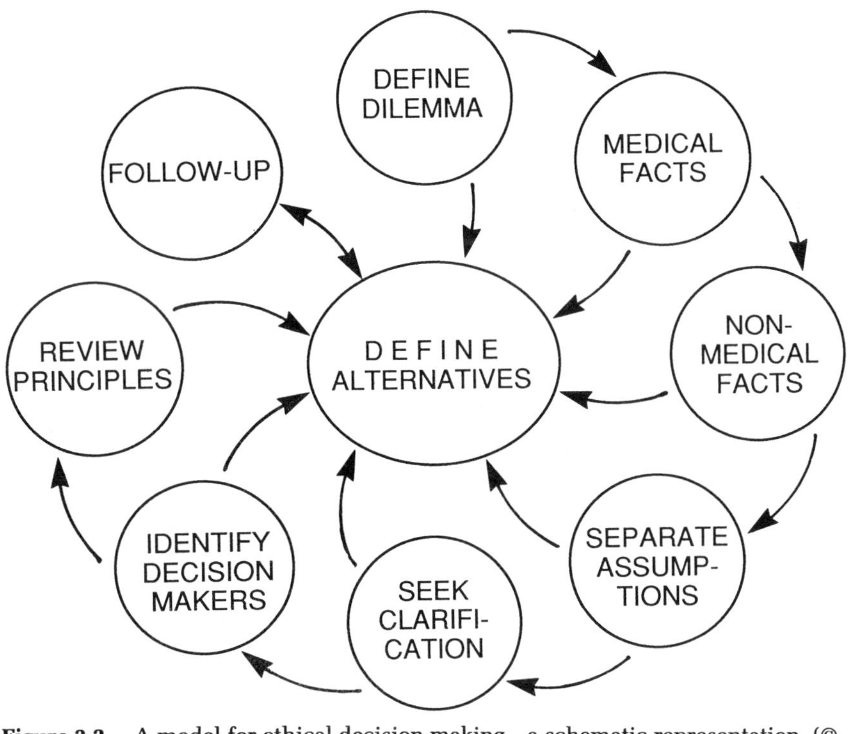

Figure 3.2. A model for ethical decision making—a schematic representation. (© Levine-Ariff, J. & Groh, D., 1987. Reprinted with permission.)

important. Coupled with a nurse's responsiveness to patient needs and preferences, right actions can be anticipated.

The use of the model as an educational tool in workshops and in ethics rounds, using either hypothetical cases or a retrospective review of actual cases, can be very valuable. Staff are then familiar with the process and able to move more quickly through the steps when confronted with an actual dilemma. Using the model for multidisciplinary ethics rounds also facilitates more open dialogue between disciplines and creates an environment in which there is greater recognition of the different perspectives of the various disciplines.

Case Examples: Clinical Case

You are a nurse in the coronary care unit. You have a 16-year-old female patient with acute bacterial endocarditis, who has been placed on *strict* bedrest. You have explained the disease process to her and the rationale for the prescribed treatment. She expresses understanding of the care plan but has repeatedly violated the order for strict bedrest. You have found her out of bed, in the bathroom or sitting in a chair, on several occasions. The attending physician, a rather traditional and authoritarian cardiologist, has stated, "If you can't keep her in bed, then put her in restraints" What do you do?

Analysis of Case Example with the Model

I. Identify the Dilemma

Some may verbalize the dilemma as "Should I restrain the patient or not restrain the patient?" Others may see it as "how to get the patient to do what's best." Still others may not have a dilemma in this situation. They may either ignore the order, continue to be frustrated with the patient, or just go ahead and restrain her.

II. Identify the Medical Facts

The patient has acute bacterial endocarditis. She has been prescribed *strict* bedrest by her physician. These are the only medical facts we have currently, from the case as presented. See section V for questions and items that need clarification.

III. Identify the Nonmedical Facts

Patient and Family. The patient is 16 years old, which may not be old enough for legal consent but is certainly old enough to be involved in assent to any decisions about her care. We do not know, from the case presented, how her family feels about this situation or how involved they are. See section V below.

External Influences. Consent laws, especially any relating to emancipated status of minors, and hospital policies on the use of restraints would be pertinent to this case. Professional codes of ethics and perhaps nursing and medical standards of care are also certainly relevant. The Code for Nurses guides us to respect patient autonomy, even when we do not agree with the patient's choices, as long as the choice is informed and freely made. As stated previously, a 16-year-old person is able to give substantial input into his or her own treatment plan ethically, if not fully legally. It may be necessary to seek additional information about the standards of care relative to this patient's diagnosis. See section V below.

IV. Separate Assumptions from Fact

Is there an assumption being made that because this patient is less than 21 years old, she does not have the right to make her own choices? Is there an assumption that this "child" does not understand what is being asked of her or what may happen if she doesn't comply? If this were a competent adult, would anyone be entertaining the notion of restraining her? Is there an assumption being made that failure to comply with the doctor's orders will absolutely result in harm? It seems that if the patient is getting upset by this order, harm may be occurring anyway. Is there an assumption being made that the healthcare team "knows what's best" for the patient?

V. Identify Items That Need Clarification

These are some of the questions that may have arisen as the first four steps of the model were followed.

Step II: How long has the patient had the disease? What was her activity level at home? What precipitated this admission? Has she had prior admissions with similar orders, and what was her compliance then? What has her compliance been with other treatment requests? What are the possible effects of her failure to comply with bedrest? What is the likelihood of complications' occurring?

Step III.A: Who comprises her family? Are they involved? What is their perspective on the situation? Do they support her actions? Can they be of help in gaining her cooperation? Has the physician spoken with them? Why does the patient keep getting out of bed? Has anyone asked her? What answer has she given? Is there something she needs or wants that, if satisfied, would gain her cooperation?

Step III.B: Is the standard of practice for this diagnosis that strict bedrest is absolutely indicated? Would another physician give a different opinion? Would it be possible to allow bathroom privileges or a bedside commode? Do we have a right to restrain this patient, ethically or legally?

Nurses must be careful that they weigh benefits and burdens carefully. The answers to all these questions must be sought before the nurse can effectively resolve the dilemma.

VI. Identify the Decision Makers

Who the decision maker is in a given situation directly relates to the dilemma identified. In this case, one dilemma identified was to restrain or not restrain. Another dilemma was how to get the patient to do what's best. In either case, it is the nurse's dilemma, and as such, the decision maker is the nurse.

VII. Review Underlying Ethical Principles

In this situation the principles involved are autonomy and beneficence/nonmaleficence. The scenario places the principles in conflict. We do not want to cause the patient harm, and we want to do good. We also want to preserve patient autonomy. Which principle we hold to be of greater importance will influence our ultimate decision. Without clarifying the assumptions and getting answers, the nurse may find herself doing the opposite of what ought to be done.

VIII. Define Alternatives

What are some of the alternatives open to the nurse? She may decide to restrain the patient and should certainly be aware of the consequences of that choice. She may decide to not restrain, regardless of what the physician says. Again, the consequences of that decision should be anticipated. She could set up a patient care conference with the physician, patient, and family to pursue the questions identified in section V and reach a decision that will be agreeable to all parties. She could suggest contracting with the patient, giving her something she wants in return for compliance with the prescription for bedrest. She may suggest an alteration of the order to reach a compromise between the physician's prescription and the patient's wishes. These are but a few of the alternatives the nurse could identify and subsequently pursue.

IX. Follow-up

Based on which alternative the nurse pursues, the follow-up will vary. If she decided to restrain the patient, there may not be any follow-up necessary. If she conducted the patient care conference, there may be multiple items that will need follow-up, still-unanswered questions, or certain information that needs validation. If an agreement was reached at the conference, it may be beneficial to reconvene the group later to determine if the solution is working to everyone's satisfaction. It may be helpful for the nurse to speak later with the physician and indicate her thoughts about how the problem was resolved by working collaboratively. This can serve to provide positive reinforcement that will carry over to the next time a similar situation may occur.

Case Example: Management Case

You are the nurse manager of the intensive care unit. You receive word from the operating room that the cardiovascular surgeon has a patient that they are unable to get off the heart-lung bypass machine, and he wants to bring the patient to the unit on extracorporeal membrane oxygen (ECMO). This is a type of technology that has never been utilized in your unit before, and your staff do not know how to manage the equipment, nor do they have an understanding of the nursing care for a patient undergoing this sort of therapy. You express concern to the surgeon, but he says, "If we don't do this, the patient will die." What do you do?

I. Identify the Dilemma

For some, the dilemma in this case may be simply stated as "What do I do?" Others may express, "Can I meet the needs of the patient but also advocate for my staff?" Again, there may be some individuals who do not find this situation to be a dilemma. They might simply do as the surgeon asks, or they may refuse to comply.

II. Identify the Medical Facts

The patient is currently in the operating room on cardiopulmonary bypass.

III. Identify Nonmedical Facts

Patient and Family. Based on the case presented, you have no facts about the patient and family.

External Influences. The Code for Nurses tells us we have a responsibility to maintain competence. In this situation, the nursing staff have no basis for being able to practice competently. At the same time, the Code states that "nurses therefore must take all reasonable means to protect and preserve human life when there is hope of recovery or reasonable hope of benefit from life-prolonging treatment." Is this a reasonable means, and is there reasonable hope of recovery or benefit for this patient? What are the standards of care for this particular intervention? Is there a way to meet those standards? Would admitting this patient be placing the nursing staff in a legally precarious position with regard to their licenses, by asking them to practice in a situation for which they are not competent? Is there a current hospital policy that would govern this situation?

IV. Separate Assumptions from Facts

Is it a fact that if this is *not* done, the patient will die? Is it an assumption that if this *is* done, the patient will live?

V. Identify Items That Need Clarification

As far as medical facts, you have little information. What is the patient's primary cardiac lesion? Was it fully repaired? Why is he continuing to require bypass? Was there an untoward event during surgery that has influenced this? With regard to the patient and family, there are many questions to be asked. Does the family know about the patient's condition? Has the physician asked their consent to do this? Do they understand the risks and benefits? Do they know that it has never been performed by the nursing staff in this unit? What has been done in the operating room when this situation occurred previously?

More information must be sought about external influences, particularly standards of care. Are there resources for the staff? Is there anyone in the institution who has the expertise, such as the neonatal unit? (ECMO is a recognized therapy for certain neonatal conditions.) Have any of the nurses had experience with ECMO at another institution? Can the perfusionist from the operating room be of assistance? What support or assistance would the physician provide? What equipment, supplies, and medications are required?

VI. Identify the Decision Makers

This is not the type of situation a nurse manager would typically decide to handle completely on her own authority. Who are the other individuals in the institution who should be involved? Nursing administrative channels, up to and including the senior nurse executive, should be utilized. Does the institution have a medical director? Possibly the chief of surgery should be involved. Does the ICU have intensivists? What is their role in this decision? The nursing staff themselves should be included in this decision. How do they feel about being asked to provide care under these conditions? What resources or support would they need to feel comfortable with the situation? In some institutions, it may be appropriate to involve the risk manager. If possible, these individuals should be convened as quickly as possible to establish who the primary decision maker is and to sort through the possible alternatives.

VII. Review Underlying Ethical Principles

In this dilemma, it would seem the primary principles in operations are those of beneficence and nonmaleficence. In an effort to do good, would harm be inflicted by applying technology that the team is not prepared to competently manage? This has been called by some the "technological imperative"—the use of technology in situations where proven benefit is doubtful and/or without knowledge of all the possible consequences. Can a nurse manager ask a nurse to deliver care under these circumstances? Fidelity, or promise keeping, is also a concern. What about the promise a nurse makes to every patient to function competently, and the promise the institution makes to patients that its employees are able to care for them safely?

VIII. Define Alternatives

One alternative is to decide that this intervention cannot be provided and the surgeon will need to wean the patient off bypass in the operating room. This alternative needs to be chosen with the understanding that the patient may die if he is indeed unable to maintain his own circulation. Another alternative is to identify the resources needed to provide ECMO in the unit and agree to provide care. However, an agreement could be made that future cases would not be handled until there is a multidisciplinary group established to look into the ongoing need for the technology and plan an appropriate program for the future. It would be important, if the latter alternative were chosen, that the nurse manager very clearly state what the needs of the nursing staff are with regard to support from the surgeon, from the intensivists, and from the perfusionist. In addition, it needs to be clear that adequate staffing hours, such as two nurses for the patient instead of one, must be provided for basic safety (this is the standard staffing for an ECMO patient).

IX. Follow-Up

After the situation has been resolved and the patient has either survived or not, the nurse manager must reconvene the group that was involved in the decision for follow-up discussion. What went well with the process? What did not go well? What questions need to be asked or actions taken for preventive ethics, before the situation occurs again? Regardless of the outcome for the patient, this must be done. Too often, if the patient has a successful outcome, it is viewed that the right decision was made, and the issue is not addressed adequately before it arises again. It does not necessarily hold true that it was the right decision or that it will be the right decision the next time. If the nurse manager does not insist on this follow-up process, it is virtually certain that no one else will, and thus will begin the slippery process of having the next situation already decided as a *fait accompli.* This type of situation may well represent one of the most difficult for nurse managers today. Often there is a feeling of being between a rock and a hard place. The manager must remember her obligations to patients, to staff, and to the institution. None of these will be well served by remaining silent or allowing the self-interests of any individual to prevail.

Summary

It should be obvious that as technological achievements progress, the frequency and complexity of ethical dilemmas are increasing for nurses, not diminishing. The anguish that accompanies these dilemmas will also not diminish. Nurses, often bearing a direct responsibility for the decisions that need to be made, have the moral obligation to be actively involved. A model is presented to aid in the decision making process for such dilemmas. Only by educating themselves in ethical theory and practicing a logical, reasoned approach to these issues will nurses be able to articulate their views and serve responsibly as advocates for the patient.

REFERENCES

Curtain, L. (1980). Ethical issues in nursing practice and nursing education. In *Ethical issues in nursing and nursing education.* (pp. 22–23, 25). New York: National League for Nursing.

Fowler, M. D. M. (1987). Piecing together the ethical puzzle: Operationalizing nursing's ethics in critial care. In M. D. M. Fowler & J. Levine-Ariff (Eds.), *Ethics at the bedside: A sourcebook for critical care nurses.* (p. 183). Philadelphia: J. B. Lippincott.

Grey-Toft, P., & Anderson, J. G. (1981). The nursing stress scale: Development of an instrument. *Journal of Behavioral Assessment, 3*(1), 11–23.

Jacobsen, S. P. (1987). Stressful situations for neonatal intensive care nurses. *The American Journal of Maternal-Child Nursing, 3*(1), 144–150.

Ketefian, S. (1981). Critical thinking, educational preparation and development of moral judgment. *Nursing Research, 30*; 98–103.

Kohlberg, L. (1976). Moral stages and moralization. In T. Likona (Ed.), *Moral development and behavior.* (pp. 31–53). New York: Holt, Rinehart, & Winston.

Langham, P. (1977). Open forum: On teaching ethics to nurses. *Nursing Forum, 16,* 221–227.

Lo, B., & Schraeder, S. A. (1981). Frequency of ethical dilemmas in a medical inpatient service. *Archives of Internal Medicine, 141,* 1062–1064.

Mitchell, C. (1981). New directions in nursing ethics. *The Massachusetts Nurse, 50*(7), 7–10.

Oskins, S. L. (1979). Identification of situational stressors and coping methods by intensive care nurses. *Heart and Lung, 8*(5), 953–960.

Smith, S. J., & Davis, A. J. (1980). Ethical dilemmas: Conflicts among rights, duties, and obligations. *American Journal of Nursing, 80,* 463–1466.

Swider, S. M., McElmurray, B. J., & Yarling, R. R. (1985). Ethical decision making in a bureaucratic context by senior nursing students. *Nursing Research, 34,* 108–112.

Ustal, D. B. (1978). Values clarification in nursing: Application to practice. *American Journal of Nursing, 78,* 2059.

Yarling, R. R., & McElmurray, B. J. (1986). The moral foundation of nursing. *Advances in Nursing Science, 8*(2), 63–73.

4

Confronting Unsafe Practice

What constitutes unsafe practice? How prevalent are acts that might be deemed unsafe or questionable? Iatrogenic illness is defined as an adverse reaction to medical therapy, surgery, or diagnostic procedure. These adverse reactions may occur as haphazard or unpredictable events, such as falls; as somewhat predictable occurrences, such as side effects from certain medications; as honest mistakes or errors in judgment; or as the result of some degree of negligence (Applegate, 1986). Studies done in 1964 (Schimmel) and 1981 (Steel, Gertman, Crescenzi, & Anderson) revealed that 20% to 36% of hospitalized patients on a medical service may suffer iatrogenic illness or complications (harm), and these are considered conservative estimates. A 1986 study (Lakshmann, Hershey, & Breslau) found that iatrogenic illness may be the actual cause of as many as 5% of the admissions to a medical service. Adar's (1982) 5-year study of a surgical service revealed that 10% of those patients suffered some degree of iatrogenic complication. Not all iatrogenic harm is preventable, nor is all of it the result of poor or sloppy practice. Certainly, in the technologically complex healthcare environment of today, there are bound to be some errors made, even by competent practitioners. Does it matter whether these situations are the result of simple human error or of incompetence? The answer may influence the action taken by the nurse manager; however, the more important question is, What happens when mistakes are discovered? What processes or mechanisms are utilized to analyze these errors and ensure that they do not occur again? Does an environment exist in which practice can be scrutinized with an intent to improve care, or are mistakes covered up for fear of retribution? Is there a sense that if errors are reported, there will be responsible follow-up to prevent recurrences, or do caregivers believe that their reports would simply be in vain? How do we routinely monitor quality of care and ensure that providers meet certain standards?

Consider the following situations:

You are the evening charge nurse on a medical/surgical unit. A nurse arrives from the "float pool" to provide assistance to your unit. As you begin to give her report, you notice that she has a strong odor of alcohol on her breath. However, she seems fully in control of herself, asks pertinent questions about the patients, and is prepared to go immediately to work.

You are the nurse manager of a pediatric unit. A resident physician comes to speak with you about one of the nurses. The physician tells you that on the previous day she witnessed a nurse striking a child who was uncooperative during his percussion and postural drainage treatment. This nurse has excellent clinical skills but has been counseled repeatedly by you for situations in which her behavior has been unpredictable and out of control. For example, she has shouted at other healthcare professionals in the patient care area, and on one occasion, she threw a piece of tubing at a respiratory therapist. These outbursts are usually in response to stress, and you have been working with the nurse to help her learn how to control her reaction to stressful situations.

You are the nurse manager of a dialysis unit. Over the past several months, many of your staff have complained to you about how a particular physician has been acting. He is frequently rude and demanding, seems very forgetful, often contradicts himself, and occasionally has slurred speech and moves as if he is in slow motion. The staff have described his behavior with the phrase "It's as if he's on medication." Today, one of the patients has a seizure while on dialysis. The nurse calls to this physician, who is at the end of the hall, but he doesn't respond. The charge nurse goes to the physician and explains what is happening, but he is still very slow to react. Once he arrives at the bedside, he seems unsure about what to do. Another physician arrives and orders various interventions, including anticonvulsants. The patient recovers, and his dialysis is completed without further problems.

Unfortunately, in actual practice, none of these scenarios is far-fetched, nor even rare. What are the obligations of nurses and physicians when confronting unsafe practices? Do managers have additional obligations, beyond those of staff nurses? What is the responsibility of the healthcare institution when these issues are brought to light?

Professional Codes of Ethics

The American Nurses' Association Code for Nurses (1985) addresses a nurse's professional responsibility when confronting unsafe practice. "The nurse acts to safeguard the client and the public when healthcare and safety are affected by incompetent, unethical, or illegal practice by any person" (p. 1). The interpretive statements go on to explain that

> as an advocate for the client, the nurse must be alert to and take appropriate action regarding any instances of incompetent, unethical, or illegal practice by any member of the healthcare team or the healthcare system, or any action on the part of others that places the rights or best interests of the client in jeopardy. (p. 6)

The Principles of Medical Ethics of the American Medical Association (AMA) (1989) state that "a physician shall deal honestly with patients and colleagues, and strive to expose those physicians deficient in character or competence, or who engage in fraud or deception (p. ix). In the AMA's Opinions on Professional Rights and Responsibilities, it is made quite explicit:

> Incompetence, corruption, or dishonest or unethical conduct on the part of members of the medical profession is reprehensible. . . . A physician should expose, without fear or favor, incompetent or corrupt, dishonest, or unethical conduct on the part of members of the profession. (Council on Ethical and Judicial Affairs of the American Medical Association, 1989, p. 36)

In addition to nurses and physicians, hospital administrators are also held to a code of ethics. The American College of Healthcare Executives (ACHE), as a professional organization, has defined for its members rules of conduct, in which they state that the healthcare executive shall "assure the existence of a process to evaluate the quality of care or service rendered (American College of Healthcare Executives, 1988, p. 19). The ACHE also includes in its Code of Ethics a set of Guidelines on Ethical Conduct for Healthcare Institutions, in which it is stated that

> healthcare institutions should have specific mechanisms or procedures to resolve conflicting values and ethical dilemmas among

patients, their families, medical staff, employees, the institution, and the community. . . . The policies and practices of health care institutions should respect the professional ethical codes and responsibilities of their employees and medical staff members and be sensitive to institutional decisions that employees might interpret as compromising their ability to provide high-quality health care. (American Hospital Association, 1988, p. 21)

Legal Requirements

In addition to being held to the ethical standards delineated by professional codes of ethics, nurses and physicians are often required legally to report incompetent practice. For nursing, some of these regulations are quite broad and require reporting of all violations of a particular state's nurse practice act, while others may be more narrow in scope and quite specific as to what must be reported. In some states, failure to report a colleague's incompetent practice may in itself be considered misconduct and form the basis for disciplinary action by the licensing board (Luckenbill-Brett & Stuhler-Schlag, 1987). Several states that have instituted mandatory reporting laws for nursing have witnessed a dramatic increase in the number of incidents that are reported. In Wyoming, this was attributed to the fact that prior to having a mandatory reporting law, directors of nursing received considerable pressure from their administrators to not report impaired nurses, due to fears about adverse publicity. The reporting law clarified who was responsible for reporting, and the directors were able to insist on reporting, once they themselves were placed at risk for failure to report (Luckenbill-Brett & Stuhler-Schlag, 1987).

Unfortunately, some data indicate that the effectiveness with which reports are dealt with at the state level is quite variable and that, historically, nurses are dealt with more harshly than are physicians (Fowler, 1986; Luckenbill-Brett & Stuhler-Schlag, 1987). A series of articles in the *Miami Herald* revealed that one-third of the states do not report disciplinary actions for physicians to the national clearing house that is supposed to keep track of unfit physicians and keep them from moving from state to state (Miller, Hiassen, & Malone, 1979). A recent study at the federal level (Ready, 1989) found that the Veterans Administration is "lax in reporting physicians it has reprimanded to the state licensing boards." Some physicians have been allowed to resign or retire before hearings are conducted on charges of incompetence and thus leave the system with no record of problems.

Just as nurses and physicians can be held ethically and legally to certain standards regarding the incompetent practices of others, there is extensive precedent for the legal responsibility of the hospital and its trustees to ensure competent practice of its employees and medical staff. A hospital has a duty to monitor and control the professional activities of its medical staff, and "the hospital itself becomes accountable to the patient if it knows or should have known . . . that the physician was not competent to practice medicine in accordance with the required standard of care" (Blaes, 1982). Hospitals usually address these issues by defining the credentialing and review processes for physicians in their medical staff bylaws.

Regulations for Accreditation

Regulations set forth by regulatory or accrediting agencies, such as the JCAHO, specify that "the nursing department/service takes all reasonable steps to maintain the optimal professional conduct and practices of its members" (Joint Commission on Accreditation of Healthcare Organization, 1989, p. 133). Adherence to this standard would be demonstrated by written policies and procedures related to ethical conduct and professional practices. Policies that address the process used to monitor and evaluate instances of substandard practice and/or unethical conduct would be included. For example, in most hospitals, patient incidents are documented on a special form, sometimes called incident reports or notification forms. These documents are usually used on the advice of insurance companies to heighten awareness of potential liability. Incidents such as patient falls, medication errors, intravenous fluid infiltrations, and decubitus ulcer formation are documented. What the nursing department then does with this information is critical in demonstrating how it deals with practice issues. Some hospitals have established a mandatory follow-up form to be utilized by nursing managers each time such an incident occurs. This establishes accountability for all nursing staff to correct problematic practice (Fig. 4.1).

Clearly, not all incidents can be prevented or are the fault of a particular nurse. For example, a mother does not watch her child closely enough, and he falls out of the crib, or medication orders are not transcribed in a timely fashion because the physician does not put the chart in the proper place after writing orders. The point is that the reporting mechanism should not just become another piece of administrative paperwork. The nurse manager should be able to differentiate specific incidents, discern trends, and identify problems with systems, procedures, and staff knowledge. The information gleaned from such

INCIDENT ANALYSIS WORKSHEET
CONFIDENTIAL
Do Not Photocopy

Unit: ________________
Date: ________________

Description of Incident (detail *all* circumstances, personnel involved, outcome of incident):

Action Taken:

Personnel Involved: 1) ________________ 2) ________________
3) ________________ 4) ________________

Are parents aware of incident: Yes ______ No ____

If so, their responses:

Documentation on chart:

Employee Progress Notes:

Signature: __________________________ Title: ____________________

Figure 4.1 Incident analysis worksheet. (Reproduced with permission from Childrens Hospital Los Angeles.)

a reporting mechanism should be used to plan education for the staff and/or revise current practices. To fully meet the defined standards, there should also be a defined disciplinary procedure to follow when substandard practice is determined to be the result of incompetence or repeated error (Joint Commission on Accreditation of Healthcare Organizations, 1987, p. 7).

Similarly, there are state and JCAHO regulations governing credentialing processes that hospitals must follow for granting and renewing practice privileges for physicians. There are also provisions in the regulations that relate to quality review mechanisms for medical practice within hospitals. These are all efforts to provide assurances to the public that physicians are qualified to practice and monitor their practice appropriately. Unfortunately, these types of credentialing processes are sometimes viewed as a mere formality, and credentials may get a "rubber stamp" rather than a meaningful review. A recent study done by the General Accounting Office (Ready, 1989) found that hospitals in the Veterans Administration (VA) system did not adequately document qualifications of physicians for the granting of practice privileges and failed to verify licensing of more than half the physicians hired between 1986 and 1988. The report concluded that because of these (and other) deficiencies, the "VA cannot guarantee that its physicians are fully qualified."

It is clear that nurses, physicians, administrators, and trustees of hospitals have ethical and legal obligations to report situations that demonstrate incompetent or unsafe practice. The following sections will explore (*a*) some causes of and contributing factors to unsafe practice and the obstacles that may prevent individuals from reporting unsafe practices, and (*b*) recommended approaches to be utilized in confronting situations of unsafe practice. Finally, some steps that managers can take to minimize, and deal with, instances of unsafe practice will be delineated.

Causes of Unsafe Practice

What are the causes of unsafe or incompetent practice? Certainly, there are cases of willfull disregard for established standards—reckless individuals who believe their own judgment to be superior to that of the rest of the professional community. More frequently, though, incompetent practice is related to a failure to keep up with the latest knowledge and scientific advances, emotional or psychological distress, stress related to work or personal problems, physical illness, or substance abuse. (See "The Impaired Professional" pg. 71.)

Nurses and physicians who do things the same way, year after year, can find themselves in a comfort zone, where new practices rarely intrude. Organizations that do not have active inservice education programs, strong quality review activities, or effective evaluation systems contribute to this sort of complacency. It may not be until something serious happens to a patient that a reevaluation of procedures and techniques is undertaken. Physical illnesses, stress, or emotional illness can sometimes cause alterations in one's ability to think clearly, make decisions, or carry out procedures that require a high degree of manual dexterity.

Complicity

Nurses are sometimes caught in the middle of a situation that they perceive to be questionable. Just because someone else made the decision or initiated the action does not alleviate the nurse's complicity in wrongdoing. Consider the following examples: In the operating room, the attending surgeon breaks sterility and goes on with the procedure. The nurse does not say anything because this particular surgeon has been so nasty when breaks in technique have been mentioned before. A resident is trying to do a lumbar puncture on a patient and has made three or four attempts without success. The nurse knows that he should not continue but does nothing to stop him. A consent is obtained by the surgeon from the patient for a heart transplant. The nursing staff know the patient has a very high risk of rejecting the organ. The risks and other aspects of treatment post-transplant were not clearly explained to the patient. The operation is allowed to take place. Allowing these situations to go unblocked would be cooperating in unsafe practice.

Conscientious Objection

A nurse can refuse to carry out an order she believes is unsafe. This is commonly done in regard to inappropriate drug dosages. In some of these situations, a physician may get angry at the nurse and do it himself. Does this remove the ethical or legal liability from the nurse? Consider this example: In a busy orthopaedic clinic, a physician ordered the nurse to give intravenous Valium to a 5-year-old child. The physician stated he did not want the child squirming during cast removal. The nurse checked the dose and realized that not only was it too high, but the indications for this drug, the route, and the common side effects seemed inappropriate in this situation. The nurse explained that to the physician, who promptly said "Give me the drug and the syringe." The nurse did so, and the physician administered the drug. After cast removal, the child's blood pressure had dropped significantly, his pulse was weak, and he was quite lethargic. The child did not suffer a respiratory or cardiac arrest, and the ultimate outcome was a positive one; however, the nurse felt a great deal of moral distress at not more actively intervening in this physician's deleterious practice (June Levine-Ariff, personal communication, 1988). Nurses can refuse to work on a nursing unit they believe is giving incompetent care or where a particular physician continues to be allowed to practice. Nurses can refuse to cooperate in questionable practices and should take active means to prevent unsafe situations. If the practice is such that the nurse will not perform the act herself, how is her conscience relieved if she allows another to carry it out? How is she fulfilling ethical and legal responsibilities to protect the patient? Nurses cannot continue to hide behind the notion of their own individual quality practice. It creates too much moral distress and perhaps ultimately, if prolonged, a loss of integrity.

Obstacles to Reporting

What are the obstacles to reporting unsafe or incompetent practice? One of the most basic is the conflict the nurse may feel between her perceived duties. She has a duty to protect the patient or future patients, but she may also feel a duty of loyalty to the team member who is practicing unsafely. To speak out would be to violate the rules of the team, or group, membership. There may be fear of ostracism by the other team members or the fear of being labeled as a troublemaker, which could impede one's own career prospects. In the past, the predominant norms for nurses were to be loyal to the institution and to the physician. Under these norms, nurses would repress what was in their own or their patients' best interests. They did not want to make trouble for the physician or the institution. As the nursing profession has become more autonomous, emphasis has shifted to the role of patient advocate, and it is clear that the nurse's first duty is always to the patient. The current Code for Nurses clearly states that "neither physician's orders nor the employing agency's policies relieve the nurse of accountability for actions taken and judgments made" (American Nurses' Association, 1985). This part of the Code emphasizes the nurse's responsibility to not cooperate in wrongdoing.

Hyland and Frapwell (1986) describe that another reason for failing to report incompetent actions may be related to anxiety over one's own practice standards; "the belief that 'there but for the grace of God go I' leads to a conspiracy of silence where the observer feels guilty about the actions of the malpracticing nurse." A survey by *RN* magazine found that many nurses decide whether to report based on the perceived severity of the error, while others choose to report based on whether they judged the error to be an honest mistake or part of a pattern of incompetence. Still others viewed that it was acceptable to not report an error if the individual who makes the error seems genuinely concerned and has learned from the mistake. Some nurses admitted that their tendency to report would be influenced by how much they liked the nurse or the doctor, but as Taylor points out, "This kind of thinking contradicts a basic tenet of nursing ethics" with regard to the nurse's obligation being first to the patient and secondarily to colleagues (Cerrato, 1988).

Another obstacle to reporting unsafe practices may be the fear of retaliation or reprisal. Whether this fear is realistic or unfounded is irrelevant. The individual's perception of danger or risk to self is the factor that will influence action. Certainly, the literature on whistleblowing is replete with instances of reprisals taken against individuals who came forward with concerns. Ideally, though, if an environment exists where legitimate concerns about practice are addressed in a responsible manner, there would be no need for whistleblowing outside the institution. (Chapter 5 explores this concept in more detail.)

Numerous reports in the literature document an individuals' reluctance to report a friend whom they know is experiencing personal problems of some sort, or whom they suspect may have a substance abuse problem. The natural loyalties to a friend and repetitive assurances that the practice will improve as soon as the problems are resolved prevent the nurse from informing appropriately. Other nurses may cover for the individual by picking up the slack in her work performance and correcting or working around mistakes. Fears that the nurse would lose her job and her license if discovered and unrealistic expectations that the individual will be able to overcome the problem on her own may also be factors. A variation on this situation may be if the nurse whose practice is in question is known to be a close friend of the supervisor. Staff members may be afraid that their concerns will be ignored or covered up.

The Impaired Professional

The term "impaired professional" is used here to refer to a healthcare provider who is unable to function according to professional standards due to the effects and influence of chemical abuse and dependency, whether related to drugs or alcohol. Conservative estimates place the incidence of alcohol or chemical dependency at 1 in 10 among the American population. Physicians and nurses are at higher risk. Various studies place the rate of substance abuse and chemical dependency in nurses at anywhere from 30% to 100% higher than in the general population (Beck & Buckley, 1983; Kabb, 1984; Leffler, 1986; O'Conner, 1985). A study in Florida (Hutchinson, 1987) revealed that 60% of cases brought to the state board of nursing for disciplinary action involved chemical dependency. Other states have reported that 75% to 90% of disciplinary actions for nurses are for impairment or drug diversion (Luckenbill-Brett & Stuhler-Schlag, 1987). A study reported by Harvard Medical School (Bensinger & Fitzpatrick, 1987) revealed that more than 30% of interns and medical students admitted to using illegal drugs within the 12 months prior to the study.

What are the indicators or warning signs for an individual with a substance abuse problem? Factors that are associated with nurses becoming impaired are a high-stress environment, personal expectations, easy access, knowledge of drugs, and peer protection (Patrick, 1984). Frequently, the first apparent signs will be problems at home, such as divorce or separation (Kabb, 1984). However, these cues encompass behavior that is outside the purview of the manager and may be difficult to assess. Changes in work behavior may occur later in the disease. Behavioral and personality changes, such as irritability, withdrawal, and isolation from other staff, may occur. Increased absenteeism or tardiness, increased errors and verbal excuses, and decreased overall work quality and quantity are also frequent cues. The individual may frequently volunteer to count narcotics. Audits of the narcotic records may reveal that this individual signs for more narcotics than other staff members. Additionally, patients may deny relief from medications charted as given or deny, in fact, ever receiving the drug (Kabb, 1984; Patrick, 1984).

Occasionally a discrepancy in narcotic records may surface before there are any suspicions about a particular individual. While in the past, individuals diverting drugs may have "watered down" the multidose vial, individual-dose injection packs make that practice more difficult, or more easy to detect. The divertor may resort to forged entries or stealing "wastage" to obtain the drugs. In one situation, an emergency room nurse made up names and recorded complete entries for nonexistent patients. This was relatively foolproof, since between 150 to 200 patients were seen daily, and all of them were in and out within a matter of hours. It was difficult for other members of the healthcare team to notice anything unusual. Routine auditing of the narcotic records and patient logs revealed the discrepancy (Donna H. Groh, personal communication, 1988).

When peers recognize that a colleague is impaired, they are frequently very reluctant to confront the issue. They hope their suspicions are wrong; they may not know how to confront the issue and may fear repercussions for the individual. In the past, most nurses reported to the state licensing board for drug abuse automatically lost their licenses. Fortunately, over the last several years, many states have begun to develop programs that can assist the impaired nurse to get help without revocation of her license. Managers have a responsibility to be informed about the regulations in their state, as well as to be aware of other resources that can be accessed to support individuals with a substance abuse problem. See the section on employee support resources on page 81 for more on this. Confronting the nurse is the ethical approach that protects the best interests of not only patients but also the individual nurse.

Confronting Unsafe Practice

Raising concerns about a colleague's practice carries certain risks and responsibilities. Before actually reporting another professional for incompetent or unethical behavior, there is a duty to fully assess the situation. The following questions can be asked to determine whether a particular incident merits reporting.

- Is the practice truly incompetent, illegal, or unethical, or is it just a practice with which you do not agree? For example, there are numerous techniques that may be utilized for inserting central venous access lines. Just because someone utilizes a technique different from the one you are familiar with does not necessarily mean the practice is unsafe.
- Would an uninvolved panel of experts view the practice as acceptable? In other words, is this something that any other prudent practitioner would do under the same circumstances? Is it within the scope of the "community standard of practice"?
- Has a patient been harmed, or does the potential for harm exist? The seriousness of the harm must be assessed. If patients are, or potentially will be, in danger, the nurse must act immediately to protect them. Sometimes nurses are swayed by the good intentions of some practitioners or the obvious "usual" competency of a particular individual. As Jameton (1984) states, "The practitioner causing harm may be competent, incompetent, well meaning, or uncaring—these considerations are not as relevant as the amount of harm."
- If the outcome were different, would the conduct seem acceptable? Inherent in the practice of healthcare, there are situations when the outcome is unfavorable, regardless of the interventions used. Are you reacting to a practice that, while perhaps unorthodox, is not unsafe, and that, had the outcome been favorable, would be lauded as innovative?

After answering these questions and deciding the practice is indeed unsafe, the nurse must then decide how to approach the problem. The first action recommended by the Code for Nurses (American Nurses' Association, 1985) is to express concern to the individual carrying out the practice. It may be that through discussion with the individual, the nurse will realize that her discomfort with the "questionable practice"was due to a lack of knowledge. If the response to confronting the concern is unsatisfactory, or if this is not an isolated incident, the next step would be to inform the supervisor. When discussing concerns of this nature with your supervisor, it is important to have your facts documented clearly. Vague and unsubstantiated claims will not be seen as credible. The old axiom of news reporting serves well here; who, what, where, and when must be factually presented.

It is important to differentiate between reporting unsafe practice internally, within the institution, and externally, to licensing boards and law enforcement agencies. Certainly, there are individual, isolated incidents that may represent a situation of unsafe practice. There needs to be a mechanism within the institution to report such incidents to the appropriate managerial personnel, with the expectation that there will be follow-up and appropriate documentation, education, or supervision provided to prevent further such incidents. Employees need to feel comfortable that they can bring situations to the manager's attention and there will be appropriate action. It should be the rare situation that would require intervention beyond that of normal institutional channels.

However, what if an incident is not an isolated situation? What if this situation is part of a pattern of unsafe incidents? What if a clear problem of substance abuse has become apparent, and the individual is unwilling to face the problem and seek treatment? These are situations in which the manager may need to go to external agencies for support in dealing with the problem. As an example, an emergency room nurse had developed a clear pattern of behavior that indicated substance abuse. Her attendance record was abysmal. She had been observed on several occasions to be very slow and sometimes unable to calculate medication dosages. She exhibited slurred speech on occasion. There was a pattern of sedative usage that did not match patient records and that corresponded to her work schedule. When confronted by the manager, she repeatedly denied there was a problem and resisted efforts to refer her to a treatment program. Eventually, in order to protect patient interests, the manager had no recourse but to report the problem to the board of nursing for investigation. In this particular example, the board of nursing had a diversion program for treatment of impaired nurses but did not necessarily take action against their license (Donna H. Groh, personal communication, 1989). It is vitally important for nurse managers to be aware of the programs and regulations in their particular state.

Nurse Manager's Responsibility

When a manager is approached by an employee with concerns about incompetent or unethical practice, what is her responsibility? What steps should be taken initially? The approach will need to be different, depending on the manager's assessment of the situation. Even if the employee bringing the concern has already asked some of these questions, the nurse manager will need to review and verify or seek answers to the following kinds of questions. Is this a new employee who is just completing orientation and may need more instruction and closer supervision? Is this a single incident that represents honest human error, or is this part of a pattern of unsafe or questionable practices? Is this an employee who has had previous performance problems? Is this a physician who is open to dialogue with nursing? Is this a physician about whom there have been prior concerns? Has a patient been harmed, and to what degree? Is the harm still occurring? Is there the potential for harm to a specific patient or to others? Are other staff members aware? Do they share the concern? Does this represent a conflict in values, and therefore perhaps raise an ethical dilemma that needs to be surfaced for discussion by the multidisciplinary team and/or the institutional ethics committee?

What if the person presenting the concern is not a nurse but a physician or another healthcare professional? At this point, the approach would not necessarily differ, although the need to ask very specific questions about what was observed and the nature of the concern is intensified. While it is important to have an environment in which no one profession is held superior to another, there may be instances when one profession is not qualified to evaluate another's practice, or when there is a territorial issue involved rather than a situation of questionable practice.

The first step for the nurse manager is generally to gather as much information as possible. Ascertain whether other staff members are aware of the issue and whether they share the concern. Read the patient's chart to see what is documented, by whom. Even if the person who presented the concern has already spoken to the individual, the nurse manager will need to address the concern to the individual herself. Certainly, if a staff nurse is the focus of concern, the nurse manager will be in a position to fully investigate the situation, discuss it with her supervisor, and decide on a course of action. The nurse manager is also the individual who is aware of the total performance of a given nurse and knowledgeable about whether this is an isolated incident or part of a continued pattern of poor practice.

The issue of justice to the employee is very critical here. The term "justice" is used in many different contexts, but here it is intended to pertain to procedural justice, fairness, or due process for the individual. It is absolutely vital for the manager to provide the opportunity for the alleged offender to state her "side of the story," as it were. Certainly, the possibility exists that the individual who reported the situation did not observe the entire incident or did not interpret events correctly or did not accurately describe the situation to the manager. It may be that there were mitigating circumstances, or that the individual recognized the error herself and intended to speak to the manager about it. The point is that it is extremely important that the manager not go into an investigation with a preconceived notion of the outcome. An investigation is intended to discover all the relevant information pertinent to a given situation. The manager must not be biased in advance about what the facts are.

Physician Concerns

If the concern centers around a physician, it is appropriate for the nurse manager to discuss the issue with him and attempt to arrive at a resolution at that level, if possible. It is best to confront these issues face to face, in a private place, rather than try to discuss the situation over the phone. Be clear and specific, and avoid taking a defensive posture. If there is not resolution, the manager should inform the physician that she will need to take the issue further and then consult with her own supervisor about the next appropriate step.

If the manager is not comfortable confronting the physician directly, she should take the issue to her own supervisor and request assistance in addressing the concern to the physician or the physician's superior. It is heartily recommended, though, that the individual be given the opportunity to respond to such concerns before they are taken elsewhere, especially if this is the first such incident. If this represents a pattern of behavior and the individual has been approached previously with no satisfactory response, it may be more reasonable to proceed directly to someone in supervisory authority.

It is perhaps worthwhile at this juncture to make note of the fact that, indeed, everyone has a boss, so to speak. Just because physicians frequently function in independent practice, that doesn't mean there is not one to whom they are accountable. As stated previously, hospitals have the responsibility of ensuring that physicians on their staff are practicing competently. Every hospital, no matter how small, must have a medical staff organization and therefore someone who is charged with responsibility for evaluating physician practice concerns. Community hospitals frequently have a designated medical director for the hospital and often for specialty areas like obstetrics, intensive care, pediatrics, and so on. In larger institutions, there may be an overall medical director or a chief of medicine and chief of surgery (as examples) who are responsible for the medical staff practicing within their department. Academic or university-affiliated institutions typically have department and division heads for each of the various specialty services.

Confidentiality

Throughout a process such as this, it cannot be overemphasized how important it is to maintain confidentiality. These types of issues have the potential to damage reputations and careers. It would be irresponsible to not exercise the utmost discretion in pursuing the situation. It is important to tell staff that, while you are going to investigate their concern and follow up as appropriate, you may not be able to share the ultimate outcome with them. Your expectation would be that the practice will be stopped, and you need to be informed if it recurs. However, specifics about what actions might be taken with the nurse or physician will be confidential.

Organizational Responses

Even when discretion is used and concerns are raised in good faith to protect patient interests, managers need to be aware of the pitfalls that may await them when confronting unsafe practice. Physicians do not usually take "criticism" well, especially from anyone outside their own ranks. Even within the medical profession, these matters are viewed as extremely delicate, and there is what frequently appears to be extreme reluctance to monitor one another's practice. Unfortunately, some nursing executives will also be unwilling to confront these issues openly and responsibly. They won't provide support or assistance and may in fact try to hush-up the situation. Managers who present such concerns may be criticized themselves—that they are lying or their facts are not accurate, that they are not acting in good faith, or that their own performance does not meet standards. They may be ostracized and feel that their own credibility in the institution is being threatened.

What happens if the manager's supervisor brushes off the incident or won't support the manager in the action she thinks is appropriate? If the manager has done her investigation properly and the facts are clear, she must be guided by the ethical standards that govern practice and that take precedence over the advice of the supervisor. The American Nurses' Association Code for Nurses (1985, p. 9) states that "neither physicians' orders nor the employing agency's policies relieve the nurse of accountability for actions taken and judgments made." The supervisor should be told that the situation must be addressed and that the manager will need to take the issue further by involving her (the supervisor's) superior.

What does the manager do if she feels that a nurse needs to be terminated, but staffing is already so short that she fears one less nurse will jeopardize patient care? The reality is that if this individual deserves to be terminated for unsafe practice, then patient care is already in jeopardy. By not taking the appropriate action, that danger will only be compounded, and the nurse manager will also be culpable. Once it is recognized that an individual's practice is unsafe, the nurse manager would be cooperating in wrongdoing if the nurse were allowed to continue to practice. There are other ways and means to use in addressing the issue of adequate staffing and allocation of nursing resources, which are examined in detail in Chapter 8 on allocation of resources. The primary concern here is to not let the issue of unsafe practice be clouded by other factors. It is simply not true that any nurse is better than no nurse.

The nurse manager may encounter the situation when she has terminated an employee with full organizational support, but subsequently there is a backlash of angry or anxious feelings from other staff members who either were friends with the terminated employee or who are upset about the short staffing that has resulted with one less nurse or who may feel guilty because they initially brought the unsafe practice to light. Staff may question the appropriateness of the action and may be openly hostile toward the nurse manager. The manager needs to anticipate what the reaction from other staff may be and take that into account when she is communicating that the terminated employee will no longer be working for the organization.

Being aware of such pitfalls in advance should not dissuade managers from pursuing concerns when appropriate but should serve to reinforce the necessity of having all the relevant facts carefully documented. Be open to and seek support from other sources in the institution, if need be. There may be specific committees that would be appropriate to hear your concerns. It is important to not approach the situation by making demands about what actions should be taken. This may convey the impression that revenge or malice is involved. The nurse manager's concern is that the practice be stopped, not what specific actions are taken with the individual practitioner.

What can be done if concerns about unsafe practices are not taken seriously, if repeated situations are ignored, even after all appropriate authorities within an institution have been alerted? This is when the situation may change. Chapter 5 deals with the subject of whistle-blowing and reviews options and outcomes for the individual practitioner facing such a dilemma.

Environmental Factors

Are there contributing factors in the environment that may foster these conditions? Can managers impact the causative factors in any way? Hospital administrators, and certainly nurse managers, have a responsibility to create an environment that not only supports the practitioner's ability to practice ethically but, in addition, provides guidelines, policies, and procedures that assist staff in knowing what is expected of them. Elements that aid in the development of such an environment were discussed in Chapter 1.

Policies and Procedures

There must be policies that define the institution's expectations about behavior and accountability for care. Practices or procedures that violate professional ethical codes and practice acts must be changed. Procedures must delineate the organizational channels to be utilized for conflict resolution, for notifying attending physicians about changes in patients' status, for handling grievances, for how to access the institutional ethics committee, and the like. There must be clear procedures for reporting errors and challenging decisions made by others. Hott (1976) reports that when a group cannot question the performance of another group, we are giving privileges to one group that can override and dominate privileges of another group.

Standards of Care

Standards of care that define the minimum level of care that *every*-patient should *always* receive must be developed for all areas and services. The extent of compliance with such standards must also be monitored on an ongoing basis. Too often, institutions develop standards that are written solely for the purpose of passing JCAHO review but are never utilized to actually monitor the care provided. Does the institution subscribe to and abide by the Patient's Bill of Rights? How is that communicated? Are patients provided with that information when they are admitted to the institution? What avenues exist for the patient to express concerns about the care he/she receives?

Systems for meaningful quality assurance activities must be developed and utilized. Too frequently, quality assurance activities are geared toward technical audits. For example, when reviewing compliance with informed consent policies, hospitals may audit technical documented elements, such as whether the consent form was properly signed and witnessed and whether there is a progress note written by the physician. Rarely is the content of the progress note evaluated, and therefore, the actual process of obtaining informed consent is not reviewed at all. A common quality assurance activity for nursing is to audit whether nurses document the patient's response within an hour after receiving medication for pain. This is, of course, important, but what about looking at the accuracy of pain assessment. Were there times the patient should have received medication but did not? Were other measures employed to minimize pain? Has there been discussion with the physician regarding the most appropriate methods of pain management for the patient? Again, the tasks tend to get more attention than the process and use of judgment—the essence of competent clinical practice. Quality review must become more oriented toward the outcomes of care. All levels of staff should participate in the process, in order to develop widespread involvement and trust in the credibility of these systems.

Nurses must serve on medical staff and hospital committees that serve to safeguard client health and safety by routinely reviewing practices. Nursing management should select their representatives on such committees. These individuals should be active voting members, with the responsibility to represent their patients and the nursing staff. Managers have a duty to their employees to assure not just a safe environment but a responsive one. The department of nursing should develop systems that specify how these representatives should communicate information back to the department. Otherwise, a cohesive approach to patient care will not be realized.

Continuing Education

Mechanisms must be provided to ensure that ongoing education is available to staff. Inservice about new equipment, procedures, drugs, and the like, must be provided *before* staff are expected to utilize them in their practice. Nurses and physicians alike must be involved in planning for new clinical programs so that everyone involved is adequately prepared to perform competently when the first patients are accepted. Programs should be coordinated on-site to provide staff with information they are expected to incorporate into their practice. Opportunities to attend seminars about current trends and advances in the field should be facilitated, at least through scheduling of time to attend, if sufficient monies are not available to pay tuition. Managers should attend seminars on different practice environments, conflict resolution, strategies to achieve change, and so on. Unit files of recent and current articles from the professional literature should be compiled so that information is readily available to staff. Many hospitals have a health science library that is open to all staff. Managers should participate actively in deciding what library resources are needed for extending the level of nursing competence at the bedside.

Employee Support Resources

Does the institution provide resources such as an employee assistance program to help troubled individuals deal with their problems? Studies have demonstrated that 85% of substance-abusing individuals can return to function effectively in the workplace with the assistance of such programs (Robbins, 1987). Providing a confidential referral service and ensuring that health insurance plans cover such services is the minimum that any institution should provide its employees. The message that the institution values its employees and takes a nonjudgmental attitude toward such situations goes a long way toward ensuring a safer practice environment.

Summary

Managers who have actively chosen to move from bedside practice to management have frequently done so from a desire to positively impact the system for healthcare delivery. The motivation to improve care, correct inefficiencies, and develop the nursing staff to a higher level of professional practice should be the primary incentive for becoming a manager. Part of the responsibility that comes with the territory is confronting situations that may impinge on these goals. While confronting issues of unsafe practice is difficult, and at times frightening, it is an aspect of management that cannot be avoided. Critical to success is being knowledgeable about ethical standards and resources for support. Managers have a level of obligation, beyond that of the staff nurse, to advocate broadly for patient safety and to pursue actions that will ensure an environment in which nursing staff can practice safely.

REFERENCES

Adar, R., Bass, A., & Walden, R. (1982). Iatrogenic complications in surgery. *Annals of Surgery, 196*(6), 725–729.

American College of Healthcare Executives. (1988). *Code of ethics.* Chicago: Author.

American Hospital Association. (1973). *Patient's bill of rights.* Chicago: Author.

American Hospital Association. (1988). *Guidelines on ethical conduct for health care institutions in American College of Healthcare Executives code of ethics.*Chicago: Author.

American Medical Association. (1989). *Principles of medical ethics.* Chicago: Author.

American Nurses' Association. (1985). *Code for nurses with interpretive statements.* Kansas City, MO: Author.

Applegate, W. B. (1986). Physician management of patients with adverse outcomes. *Archives of Internal Medicine, 146;* 2249–2252.

Beck, M., 7 Buckley, J. (1983). Nurses with bad habits. *Newsweek,* Aug. 22, p. 54.

Bensinger, P. B., & Fitzpatrick, S. B. (1987). Facing up to substance abuse. *Health Management Quarterly, Third Quarter.* 9–11.

Blaes, S. M. (1982). Hospital trusteeship: Corporate and personal liability. *Hospital Progress, July,* 78–86.

Cerrato, P. L. (1988). What to do when you suspect incompetence. *RN, Oct.,* 36–41.

Council on Ethical and Judicial Affairs of the American Medical Association. (1989). *Current opinions on professional rights and responsibilities.* Chicago: Author.

Fowler, M. D. (1986). Doctoring or nursing under the influence. *Heart and Lung, 15*(2), 205–207.

Hott, J. R. (1976). The struggles inside nursing's body politic. *Nursing Forum, 15*(4), 325–340.

Hutchinson, S. A. (1987). Chemically dependent nurses: Implications for nurse executives. *Journal of Nursing Administration, 17*(9), 23–29.

Hyland, M., & Frapwell, C. (1986). Afraid to tell. *Nursing Times, Oct. 1,* 50–51.

Jameton, A. (1984). *Nursing practice: The ethical issues.* Englewood Cliffs, NJ: Prentice-Hall.

Joint Commission on Accreditation of Healthcare Organization. (1987). *Hospital accreditation program scoring guidelines for nursing services.* Chicago: Author.

Joint Commission on Accreditation of Healthcare Organization. (1989). *Accreditation manual for hospitals.* Chicago: Author.

Kapp, G. M. (1984). Chemical dependency—helping your staff. *Journal of Nursing Administration, 14*(11), 18–23.

Lakshmann, M. C., Hershey, C. O., & Breslau, D. (1986). Hospital admissions caused by iatrogenic disease. *Archives of Internal Medicine, 146;* 1931–1934.

Leffler, D. (1988). Addicted nurses—how you can lend them a helping hand. *Nursing Life, May/June,* 41–43.

Luckenbill-Brett, J. L. & Stuhler-Schlag, M. K. (1987). Mandatory reporting: Legal and ethical issues. *Journal of Nursing Administration, 17*(12), 32–38.

Miller, G., Hiassen, C., & Malone, D. (1979). Dangerous doctors. *Miami Herald* series of articles from Feb. 2 to March 4.

O'Conner, P. (1985). Managing impaired nurses. *Nursing Administration Quarterly, 9*(2), 2.

Patrick, P. K. S. (1984). Self-preservation: Confronting the issue of nurse impairment. *Journal of Substance Abuse Treatment, 1,* 99–105.

Ready, T. (1989, Sept. 11). Study: VA fails to probe doctors' histories. *Healthweek,*p. 9.

Robbins, C. E. (1987). A monitored treatment program for impaired health care professionals. *Journal of Nursing Administration, 17*(2), 17–21.

Schimmel, E. M. (1964). The hazards of hospitalization. *Annals of Internal Medicine, 60,* 100–110.

Steel, K., Gertman, P. M., Crescenzi, C., & Anderson, J. (1981). Iatrogenic illness on a general medical service at a university hospital. *New England Journal of Medicine, 304*(11), 638–642.

5

Whistleblowing

The world is full of fearful people
Trying to run away from themselves
Their thoughts roaming lazily
Through the changeless gardens
Of the past—
Not in search of data
To serve the present
But in an ineffectual attempt
To escape the insistent claims
Of this moment.

—B. Shank

Imagine you are the nurse manager in one of the following scenarios. As you read, consider the following questions: Would you report the incident? To whom? What if you received no feedback or unsatisfactory answers? What if the incident happened again? What if you were told to say nothing more about the incident?

- It was a routine occurrence in the emergency room that when patients died, the resident staff used them to practice intubation. Nurses consistently complained to the head nurse, who agreed with their concerns. She told the staff the medical director had promised to minimize this activity. But he stated, "After all, do you want the residents practicing on live patients?"
- Over the past year, a number of children had fallen out of their cribs

due to faulty locking devices. All incidents were documented through official hospital channels. One child had been seriously injured. There was no way to repair the cribs. The nursing department estimated that the hospital would need to replace all of the cribs at a cost of $250,000. A year had been spent documenting incidents. The hospital administrators kept saying they were trying to get the needed money.

- A nurse manager reported to her supervisor that she suspected a physician was sexually abusing his patients. The nurse manager had a report from one nurse who had witnessed behavior indicating such activity. Two weeks later the nurse manager was informed about Dr. Samson's "behavior." She again reported the incident to her supervisor, who thanked her again for the information. The nurse manager asked the supervisor if there had been any action since the last report. The supervisor stated that the medical director and director of nursing had been notified.

Whistleblowing

Whistleblowing became more prominent in the 1960s, as an outgrowth of the consumer and civil rights movements. In a telling exposé, Ralph Nader portrayed the stories of whistleblowers from various industries. Drs. John Gofman and Arthur Tamplin, employees of the Atomic Energy Commission (AEC), publicly expressed concern about the effects of radiation from nuclear power plants. Edward Gregory, safety inspector at General Motors, played a major role in callbacks of 1965–1969 models of Chevrolet cars due to faulty exhaust systems. Dr. Jacqueline Verett reported publicly on her research with cyclamates. Her report facilitated the Food and Drug Administration recalls. All four individuals had expressed their concerns internally on repeated occasions (Nader, Petkas, & Blackwell, 1972).

The term "whistleblowing" is used to refer to the action taken when an employee goes outside the organization to call attention to internal negligence or to dangers that have, or potentially will, threaten individuals. No other word aptly describes the circumstances in which an individual finds it necessary to report externally on problematic internal issues. The whistleblower goes outside the organization to report wrongdoing because the internal organization is seen as either ineffective or a dangerous place to share information.

Threats to patient safety may come from prescribed treatments, environmental hazards, staffing inadequacies, or the illegal or unethical conduct of any professional. Employees, especially nurses, are among the first to recognize unsafe practices, adverse effects of new technology and drugs, discriminatory practices, and diversions of drugs or supplies. They are often the first to identify actual or potential hazards within the work environment.

As employees and professionals, nurses are often caught between the values and norms of the institution and the values and standards of the profession of nursing. As professionals, nurses discuss the need for commitment to an ethical standard of practice. The Code for Nurses stresses responsibility to the patient and public and states that "the nurse acts to safeguard the client and public when health care and safety are affected by incompetent, unethical, or illegal practice of any person" (American Nurses' Association, 1985).

As employees, nurses are held to standards of loyalty and/or support for others. The institution's needs are expected to, and often do, take precedence over professional concerns. The nurse can be compromised both ethically and legally. For example, an occupational health nurse is aware of a large number of employees complaining of symptoms indicative of chemical toxicity. The nurse has repeatedly reported her concerns to management. Public exposure of this situation would significantly increase company expenditures and decrease profits. Predicted financial impact would occur from acquiring new equipment, increased medical claims, and adverse publicity. These potential adverse effects on the organization may inhibit some professionals from adhering to responsibilities. By not reporting her concerns, the nurse is not fulfilling her moral responsibilities to her patients and, in this situation, certainly not complying with state and/or federal regulations for reporting such environmental hazards.

Loyalty is defined as uncritical support of and adherence to values, norms, and practices of the group. For that loyalty, the employee continues to have a job, get pay increases, and sometimes gains status and power. "Human error" is considered acceptable among the group members, sometimes seeming to have no boundaries or limits. Adherence to this internal "code" reinforces and rewards individuals who don't tell "secrets" about things that happen inside the organization. Behaviors that threaten group norms are punished with rejection or abandonment, temporarily or permanently.

"No one enjoys admitting a mistake—especially one that has harmed a patient" (Greenlaw, 1982, p. 81). Nurses face the possibility of witnessing others' mistakes and potentially being "ordered" to cover up those mistakes. Pressure to conform comes from both supervisors and peers, putting an individual nurse in a difficult situation.

To win the nurse's sympathy to comply with the order, loyalty to the individual and/or the institution is evoked. Many nurses actually believe that failure to comply with the cover-up may be reasonable grounds for disciplinary action. Even when nurses know that it is wrong to falsify a medical record and thus not bring the error to light, they follow the order. The incident may not be pursued, even when nurses recognize that they themselves may be found at fault for the act. They often do not believe that "the consequences of the cover-up are usually worse than what it seeks to conceal" (Greenlaw, 1982, p. 82).

Legally, failure to report activities such as these is negligence by omission. In a number of cases, nurses failed to pursue a physician who ignored their repeated reports that his patient was suffering from serious problems. The nurses were found guilty by omission for failing to report negligence on the part of the physician (Regan, 1982; *Toth v. Community Hospital of Glencove,* 1982; *Utter v. United Hospital Center, Inc.,* 1977). The Code for Nurses promotes a higher response than to oneself or one's employer, making promises to the public to safeguard patient welfare. The nurse is judged by the standard of what another reasonable and prudent nurse would do under the same circumstances.

Why are individuals reluctant to push the system in order to right wrongs? Why are there so few accounts in the literature of whistleblowing by healthcare providers? It may be that whistleblowing seems so repugnant because the person doing the whistleblowing is considered to be a traitor (squeal, informer, muckraker, stool pigeon) to the team. The other members of the group may feel betrayed.

It is true, however, that "few situations present a clear, undeniable wrong—or a clear undeniable way to proceed" (Price & Murphy, 1983). Even when some situations foster outright indignation at the way people are treated, or the response of the organization to serious problems, some individuals do not know where to begin. They fear reprisals and do not know how to protect themselves or their patients. Unfortunately, some of these individuals leave the profession and/or suppress the injustices. Blowing the whistle requires energy and thoughtful investigation. It is important to assess the situation and understand that there is work to be done before going outside the organization (Fig. 5.1). Chapter 4, on unsafe practice, discusses this in more detail.

AN APPROACH TO WHISTLEBLOWING

1. Know your own values
2. Gather the facts
3. Identify the ethical concern(s)
4. Assess the environment
5. Identify the legal issues
6. Identify the internal resources
7. Identify the external resources

Figure 5.1. An approach to whistleblowing. (© Levine-Ariff, J. 1988. Reprinted with permission.)

An Approach to Whistleblowing

Know Your Own Values

Does your concern reflect how you would want to be treated? In a clinical situation, find out the patient's preference, and see if the patient, or the surrogate decision maker, has made his/her desires known. The nurse can help the patient or family convey their wishes to the appropriate individual(s). Institutional issues must be looked at in the same way. When protesting an organizational problem, an employee must be sure that the protest does not come on the heels of her having been disciplined or adversely impacted; otherwise, the nurse's motives will be in question. The motive for alleging misconduct or abuse must be above suspicion. The nurse must make sure that she is acting out of concern for others' interests, unless, of course, the nurse could be personally harmed by the situation. This approach will enhance credibility.

Gather the Facts

Sometimes, in the heat of passion, good judgment is not exercised. It is not uncommon for assumptions to be stated as fact. Be sure to check out all the data. The burden of proof is usually on the whistleblower. "Dissent demands accuracy and rational judgment" (Murphy, 1981). Accurate and complete information is always a precondition to contacting outside agencies. Make sure you can state in specific terms what is wrong, why it is wrong, and who is being or could be harmed. Take the example of a patient who tells a nurse that a certain doctor makes unwelcome advances. The nurse may become incensed at this situation and want to immediately correct the situation. There may, in fact, be a serious problem, but unless the nurse is willing to ask the patient some very specific questions, the nurse will not be treating anyone fairly. She must find out what the patient said and did when the physician approached. What exactly did the physician do and say? How often did these occurrences happen? All information that would support the accusations must be collected and documented. It is important to remember that in most cases of whistleblowers, they did not publish classified material or appropriate other documents to substantiate their claims. They simply spoke the truth, backed up by accurate and reliable data.

Identify the Ethical Concerns

Define who or what is threatened and the severity of the harms that are present or may result. Clarify how far the situation has deteriorated. Is the problem just arising, or has it existed for a long time? Is there immediate danger to the individual? Will a delay cause significant harm? How can blowing the whistle be protective? This lends objectivity to a potentially explosive situation.

Is there something that the nurse can do immediately to protect the patient(s) from further harm? The Miofsky case in 1982 is a clear example of nurses failing to actively intervene with a physician's known sexually abusive behavior with vulnerable patients. The nurses had internally reported this situation to their supervisor. Other nurses and physicians knew about the unethical and illegal behavior. The court stated,

> In their respective positions of authority at the hospital Dr. O'Kane and Nurse O'Kane each owed the patients a fiduciary duty which in addition to protection of the patients, is a duty to make full and fair disclosure of all facts which materially affect their rights or interest. It cannot be seriously contended that Miofsky's activities did not materially affect the rights and interest of the patient victims. By suppressing the information concerning Miofsky these accused health care providers breached their fiduciary duties towards those patients that had been victims. (*O'Kane v. Board of Registered Nursing,* 1982).

Assess the Environment

Assess whether your concerns are shared by other nurses or other healthcare professionals. Find out if anyone else has protested a similar situation. When serious patient care issues arise, collective action may be helpful to minimize individual consequences. It is also more difficult to ignore a group of individuals. It may be important to have to corroboration of others if charges are being brought against individuals who have substantial power in the organization. However, whistleblowers usually do their talking by themselves. Many people, even knowing what is going on, do not speak up and may even be participating in those activities. In the situation described above, the nurse also must find out whether other allegations have been made about this physician. If the patient denies the story, the facts will be difficult to substantiate without other instances of this behavior. It is usually at this point in the process that a nurse will decide whether or not to pursue the issue—whether she has enough of a case to proceed.

Identify the Legal Issues

Are laws or regulations being violated? The nurse should be knowledgeable about the state nurse practice act and any subsequent board of nursing positions. The California Board of Registered Nursing, in 1985, adopted a position that the failure of a registered nurse to report known or suspected instances of client abuse, physical, emotional, or sexual, constitutes unprofessional conduct and is grounds for discipline by the Board (California Board of Registered Nursing, 1987). This type of position is consistent with the Board's role in ensuring minimum standards of safe care for the public. Sometimes that information, highlighted in a conversation to the responsible manager, can change the course of events by making people aware of information they did not previously have.

Identify the Internal Resources

Be open to support. "Courage can be contagious" (Lippitt, 1983, p. 89). Individuals within the organization hierarchy, specific committees, and the like, may be appropriate listeners to your concerns. If possible, start with normal bureaucratic channels and keep going up the chain of command. Select those who have the power to investigate your concerns and perhaps protect and support you. Know the committee structure well enough to recognize which committee should be approached. The name of a committee can be misleading. Ask questions; find out about normal agenda items and who the members of the committee are. Approach either the chairperson or a committee member. Who you know and what the topic is may guide your decision. If you are told that the problem is being looked into or remedied, give the system a chance to work, as long as danger isn't imminent. Clarify when you can expect feedback. Emphasize your concerns. Remember, your aim is to stop a certain situation from continuing, not to punish someone.

To go public, one should be able to prove clear and imminent danger to an individual or individuals. This has certainly been true of whistleblowers in the automobile industry, the Food and Drug Administration, and the Atomic Energy Commission. However, in hospitals, sometimes the danger has already occurred, such as a death in the operating room that occurred because the wrong anesthetic agent was used, or a patient's suffering severe complications because of an inappropriate drug order. These types of situations demonstrate retrospective harm and must be reported to the appropriate internal authorities. These acts would not necessarily lead to whistleblowing unless attempts were made to cover up the incidents or they kept being repeated. Whistleblowers go public when the internal systems of an organization attempt to stifle questioning or lack an organized approach to settle differences.

Sandra Bardenilla, a staff nurse at Kaiser Hospital in Harbor City, California, inquired at the Los Angeles County Coroner's office about the stated cause of death for Mr. Clarence Herbert. Ms. Bardenilla, after repeated unsuccessful internal efforts to clarify the circumstance surrounding the withdrawal of food and fluids from Mr. Herbert, called the coroner's office. The coroner, concerned about the inquiry, contacted the district attorney's office, which indicted Drs. Nigel and Barber for the murder of Mr. Herbert. The charges were subsequently dismissed, after a thorough investigation (Steinbock, 1983). The adverse publicity that ensued for the nurse, the doctors, and the hospital caused a severe public mistrust of all healthcare professionals and institutions. Physicians and hospitals, concerned with the risk of liability, curtailed the use of withholding and/or withdrawing life-sustaining treatments. The pain and suffering experienced by the nurse and the two physicians could certainly have been avoided in an environment that promoted collegiality between all professionals and encouraged open discussion about patient care concerns.

Identify the External Resources

Nurses may seek legal counsel for personal information and/or protection. Litigation is expensive, time consuming, and emotionally draining. It may also not bring the desired results. However, nurses have used this route with some positive outcomes. Witt reported the events that ultimately led to her whistleblowing and subsequent termination. She sued the hospital for reinstatement, compensatory damages, and punitive damages. Two years later, after a failed appeal attempt by the hospital, she is awaiting the setting of damages (Witt, 1983). Margaret Rookard, director of nursing at Harlem Hospital in New York, was terminated for refusal to sign permits for foreign nurses who did not work for her. She won the right, under a federal court of appeals, to challenge her dismissal on First Amendment grounds. (Public employees who are dismissed for speaking out on matters of public interest may have a claim under the First Amendment of the United States Constitution; *Rookard v. Health and Hospitals Corp.*, 1982.)

At this point, legal advice can give the nurse information regarding some states' whistleblowers' protection laws. Michigan and Connecticut have pioneered such laws. In April 1989 President Bush signed into law a bill that prevents federal employees from disclosing the names of whistleblowers and makes it easier for federal employees to prove retaliation against them (Means, 1989).

Union contracts may limit certain management firing prerogatives. Most contracts have a "just cause" provision that requires managers to have well-documented evidence for terminating employees. In the absence of a written employment agreement, employees can be terminated at the will of the employer or employee. Although this provision exists in current labor codes, many exceptions exist. For example, the National Labor Relations Act (NLRA) protects various union-related activities; the federal Civil Rights Act of 1964 forbids discharge because of race, color, religion, sex, national origin, pregnancy, childbirth, and related medical conditions. Some states have separate statutes that protect employees engaged in various activities from discrimination or discharge. Some of the protected activities in California, for example, are jury duty, labor or political activity, the right to not participate in abortions, and submission of reports to the authorities regarding patients who appear abused or neglected (Cal. Labor Code 52301; Cal. Labor Code 1101–1105; Cal. Health and Safety Code 25955 (a); Cal. Government Code 29401e). The New York legislature, in 1983, passed an amendment to the labor law supporting a section on the rights of professionals to refuse to participate in activities that may constitute professional misconduct (Feliv, 1983). Additionally, many state courts have upheld that an employee may not be discharged for refusing to participate in illegal or questionable acts (*O'Sullivan v. Mallon*, 1978; *Pierce v. Ortho Pharmaceutical Corp.*, 1980; *Tameny v. Atlantic Richfield Co.*, 1980; *Trombettea v. Detroil*, 1978). Generally, these types of cases have fallen into a public policy exception to the "at-will" rule. Courts define the issue of public policy in different ways. The difficulty presented by all these cases is for the court to determine what is or is not contrary to public policy.

Understanding under what conditions individuals can be terminated and following careful documentation procedures are essential. Common law protection for whistleblowers is growing, yet predictable outcomes for cases are uncertain. A strong moral basis may still be found to have weak legal footing (Tobias, 1989; Meyerowitz, 1985).

Contacting a professional association (of which the nurse is a member) may provide information and/or support. The purpose of a professional association is to advance the professional goals. The association may attempt direct contact with the employer or help the nurse to publicize the case. The association would then have the same responsibility as the employee. Ralph Nader suggested the professional societies develop mechanisms to censure employers that ignore the ethical obligations of its members. Charles Petter reported that the American Society of Civil Engineers has tried to clear his name with potential employers (Nader et al., 1972). Both the American Nurses' Association and the American Association of Critical Care Nurses (AACN) have adopted statements delineating a process for addressing current ethical issues (Committee on Ethics, 1985; Ethics Committee, 1985). Certainly, they have been known to expose unsafe practice environments causing real or potential harm to patients.

Blowing the Whistle

Before blowing the whistle, the nurse needs to know who to contact. Will a state or federal agency be the most appropriate place? It would be important for the nurse to investigate the function of different agencies, who they report to, and what their usual procedures are. Should the newspaper be immediately contacted? What individual on which newspaper should be contacted?

Anonymously leaking the information to the media can be less dangerous for the whistleblower. The informer "Deep Throat" who leaked information during Watergate has never been absolutely identified. In Philadelphia, a joint state and federal inquiry was initiated by letters from an anonymous group of employees who alleged that "outrageous medical and surgical practices" had occurred at the hospital and "had resulted in unnecessary injury or death to many patients" (Stecklow, 1988).

But there are problems with leaking information. The information can be used haphazardly and possibly irresponsibly. Because the individual chooses to remain anonymous, the credibility of the information may be diminished. Like gossip, as the story gets told and retold, it can became quite distorted. Some organization do recognize the risks inherent in whistleblowing and have instituted mechanisms for employees to report information anonymously. For example, Los Angeles County instituted a "tattler hot line" that is staffed by individuals from the auditor-controllers office (*Los Angeles Times,* 1988). Organizations that institute such procedures encourage employees to report harmful situations. Organizations then have an obligation to investigate any allegations swiftly and fairly.

Be Realistic About the Chances for Success

Blowing the whistle involves risks, both personal and professional. "A risk is simply the act of seeking to achieve a goal that exceeds usual limits" (Kirk, 1986). Institutional policies, laws, unwritten rules, and administrative decisions may make adherence to responsibility difficult and thus ask us to take risks. This guarantees neither correction of the ill nor protection against reprisal. Some individuals avoid risks, and some confront them. There is no disagreement that blowing the whistle can involve risks for the nurse. The Code for Nurses does not expect the nurse to risk her own life for the life of a patient. However, knowing about and/or participating in activities that harm patients is not ethically or legally condoned. Attempts to correct the wrongdoing may not be successful. But it does not necessarily follow that the individual should not have brought the issue to light.

When delay may result in great harm, the nurse must assume the authority that she has by not following certain orders, physically protecting the patient, going to the top of the organization immediately, and/or going outside the organization. Professionals cannot always close their eyes. Nader writes that whistleblowing is an expression of the fundamental liberties of a free society. Whistleblowing has saved lives, and prevented injuries, abuse, disease, corruption, waste, and exploitation of vulnerable persons and the environment (Nader et al., 1972).

The Consequences

A physician will not be disciplined for refusing to perform a procedure for which he is not competent or to which he has moral objections. Refusing to engage in activities that compromise patient care may be seen as commendable and heroic. The problem of maintaining professional integrity is far more difficult for nurses. Consequences for refusing to participate in such activities or reporting them can be far more serious. Consequences have included ridicule, social ostracism, economic loss, and personal and professional harassment. Demotions, firings, and blacklisting have also occurred. Attacks on one's competence and judgment can occur. When Gofman and Tamplen spoke, they had little support within the AEC, and within the scientific community. Attacks centered on their style, loyalty, and motives—everything except the real issue. Their passion and zeal were critical. As their challenge grew stronger, so did the opposition. Their only choice was to submit in silence or renew their challenge in even stronger terms. Their success may have been due to the course they took (Nader et al., 1972). Witt, although she ultimately saw the truth exposed about patient abuse at the psychiatric facility where she worked, suffered termination, attacks on her mental state, and questioning of her professional competence.

It is too easy to stifle criticism and the moral consciousness of employees by an appeal to authority—by rendering them unable to "defy the bureaucracy." The very qualities that make for effective and contributing employees are often seen in individuals who whistleblow. Frank Camps, an engineer with Ford Motor Company, was directly involved in the development of the Ford Pinto. He publicly denounced the safety of the automobile. "Had Camps been treated as a voice to be heeded rather than a protester to be ignored and punished, Ford might have avoided fatalities and serious injuries, years of litigation, and the stigma of corporate irresponsibility" (Glazer, 1983).

Ultimately, suppression tactics are self-defeating for any organization. It can make martyrs of its victims and rally their allies. It will discourage internal self-correction. It gives a message to managers that it is better to ensure conformity and adherence to the rules. Myron Glazer (1983) describes three distinct paths whistleblowers tend to take: (*a*) Unbending resisters protest within the organization. They maintain a strict commitment to their principles. Ultimately, due to retaliation within the organization, they take a public stand. (*b*) Implicated protesters speak out within their organizations but acquiesce when they are ordered to conform. They find themselves drawn into illegal or unethical behavior, which they eventually expose when they fear legal liability. (*c*) Reluctant collaborators become deeply involved in acts they privately condemn. They seek remedies only when they leave the organization.

When cover-ups are honored and internal abuses continue, the healthcare provider who whistleblows faces the public not only discussing the issue but sometimes defending his/her profession, institution, and often the entire healthcare community. Situations revealing such practices erode the relationship of trust between the patient and the healthcare professional. Consider the feelings that probably arose in the jury when the nurse in the book *The Verdict* (Reed, 1980) finally came forth and testified that she had falsified hospital records to protect a physician and her job. The judgment of all nurses and the safety of all hospitals was clearly in question.

The Internal Environment

Within the ethical, professional, and legal restraints to which all of us are subject, we can and must create a system that allows for respectful dissent and conscientious objection" (Curtin, 1983). An environment must be maintained in which nurses can disagree with established procedures and/or refuse to render service. Institutional policies must provide structure to do so. Each institution providing nursing services has an obligation to have an established process for the reporting and handling of practices by individuals or healthcare institutions that jeopardize client health and safety. The conflict between loyalty to an institution and duties to the patient will surely arise.

Nursing management must take effective and preventive measures to ensure that the system encourages, not stifles, advocacy behavior. When employees have to go outside the system to correct wrongs, management is usually at fault. Some things that can be done to prevent whistleblowing and, more important, to prevent the need for whistleblowing are the following:

- Utilize clear policies for documenting violations of practices and policies.
- Design appropriate protection for those who report; confidentiality must be ensured.
- Ensure no cover-ups. The person who made the report should be kept informed of the investigation.
- (For the nurse manager:) Help the nurse(s) use the appropriate mechanism to report. In one situation, nursing staff in the operating room wrote a petition to the chief of surgery stating they would not continue to work with a particular physician. Although the nursing staff had reported this surgeon's behavior a number of times, the nurse manager just kept reporting the incidents to the head of surgery. The nurse manager failed to recognize the severity of the surgeon's behavior and the intensity of the nurses' concern. What resulted was an angry nurse manager, chief of surgery, and surgeon, with no issue resolution. Subsequently, the chief nursing executive

stepped in and met with all involved. She listened to the issues and asked the operating room nurses to state how they expected this surgeon to act. She relayed this to the chief of surgery, explaining the seriousness of the surgeon's behavior and that unless the behavior changed, there could be difficulty staffing his cases. The nurse executive asked the nurses to document future incidents in a specific way and told them to whom to forward their concerns. She also discussed with the nursing staff the options available, should this situation or similar ones arise with any healthcare provider. The valuable lesson that the nursing executive taught was not just what to do in situations with this surgeon, but how to deal with like situations. Anticipatory planning is necessary so that individuals have some control over their professional environments and thus foster a more open atmosphere.

- Support the individual who reports abuses or unsafe situations. When staff have the courage to report a certain situation, it is management's responsibility to attempt to protect that individual from adverse peer group reaction. Sometimes the group reaction is subtle. The nurse manager can verbally let the "group" know that behavior that interferes with the nurse's performing her role safely will not be tolerated. Should such behavior occur, the nurse manager must act swiftly with appropriate disciplinary action. The contemplation of such action should be discussed with the staff. Perhaps then such adverse reactions can be minimized or eliminated.
- Maintain knowledge about laws and regulations that govern hospitals. Much of the whistleblowing in private and governmental industry arose from noncompliance with industry standards. Much of the whistleblowing in healthcare appears to have arisen from a lack of adherence to accepted professional standards of patient care.
- Do not deny that managers or the organization make mistakes; to do so is to contribute to a future of many more mistakes. Open discussion creates an atmosphere of trust and promotes cooperation. It gives the manager an opportunity to explain the organization's position on why something occurred and what is being done to correct the situation.

Until management views employees as individual, responsible citizens, workers will continue to have difficulty objecting internally to unsafe products, environmental hazards, and dangerous patient care situations. It is only within an open atmosphere that ethical questions can be raised, principles clarified, and various alternatives outlined. Nursing management must place itself in a leadership role to explore with its colleagues the development of mechanisms that will encourage open dialogue about current and future ethical concerns.

Summary

As Leah Curtin said, "Perhaps there never were any 'good old days' when people knew what they ought to do and did it. And were respected for doing it" (Curtin, 1986). All nurses have an obligation to themselves and to their patients to recognize and give voice to the ethical dilemmas they confront. The American Nurses' Association's Code for Nurses does not condone ethically passive behavior (American Nurses' Association, 1985).

Nursing managers have an obligation to ensure that the channels of hierarchical communication work efficiently. All nurses have an obligation to themselves and to their patients to utilize those channels. Environments that support the status quo, stifle open discussions, and support the dominance of any profession over another will not be clinical settings where patient care is optimal. Nurses will be encouraged to seek solutions to internal ethical issues through external means: governmental agencies, newspapers, and legal action, to name a few examples.

It is incumbent upon each nurse to recognize that ethical decision making is a slow and sometimes difficult task. Ethical dilemmas are not easily solved. There are no set rules or formulas that will guarantee a successful outcome. One correct "solution" rarely exists. There are no simple answers or resolutions to issues that could lead to whistleblowing. Thus going outside the internal organization to report abuses should be done reluctantly and cautiously. What alternatives should be pursued? Who should be notified? What should be said? When should something be said? These questions should be asked and answered early. Consequences should be anticipated, yet not all outcomes can be identified.

Evidence from Glazer (1983) and Nader (1972) support the fact that there is life after whistleblowing. Individuals have rebuilt lives and often have gone on to more successful and fulfilling careers. But the human and financial costs cannot be minimized. For example, Joseph Rose (who became aware of illegal political payments to the Nixon re-election campaign) testified against his employer, Associated Milk Producers. Blackballed from employment for 8 years, as of 1983, Mr. Rose is now a successful San Antonio attorney (Nader et al., 1972). Sandra Bardenilla won a lawsuit for wrongful termination against Kaiser Hospital (Stevens, 1988).

With such potential for adversity, why would anyone undertake such actions? Living with knowing what is happening is difficult for many individuals. For nurses, it is especially difficult if patients are being significantly harmed. Ultimately, it is up to the individual, alone with his/her conscience, to report abuses. "Whether or when someone will blow the whistle will depend on the peculiar mixture of sustenance and punishment, as well as the person's courage and circumstances of his or her life" (Nader et al., 1972). John Gofman, when asked if he would speak out again, stated, "Where the future of the human species is at stake, be sure your voice is loud enough and incisive enough to be heard well" (Nader et al., 1972). Christine Spahn Smith, deserted by colleagues and "punished" by her employer for speaking up about potential patient care abuses, stated, "I would not have done anything differently" (Smith, 1980).

Some individuals, like Karen Silkwood (a nuclear plant worker who revealed flawed safety procedures) and Frank Serpico (the New York City policeman who testified about corruption) have become American folk heroes. However, it must be obvious that most whistleblowers are ordinary people upholding professional and/or personal values. They are not heroes or even individuals who always spoke up. They were, however, convinced that their beliefs should not be compromised.

REFERENCES

American Nurses' Association. (1985). *Code for nurses with interpretive statements.* Kansas City, MO: Author.

California Government Code (29401e).

California Health and Safety Code 25955 (a).

California Labor Code S2301.

California Labor Code 1101-1105.

Committe on Ethics. (1985). *Guidelines on mechanisms through which state nurses' associations consider ethical issues and concerns.* Kansas City, MO: American Nurses' Association.

Curtin, L. (1983). A nurse's conscience. *Nursing Management, 14* (2); 8.

Curtin, L. (1986). Sister Angelique "blows the whistle." *Nursing Management, 17*(10), 7–8.

Ethics Committee. (1989). *Process for addressing current ethical issues.* Newport Beach: American Association of Critical-Care Nurses.

Feliu, A. G. (1983). Thinking of blowing the whistle. *American Journal of Nursing, 83,* 1541–1542.

Greenlaw, J. (1981). What to do if your supervisor orders a "cover-up." *RN,* Oct., 81.

Glazer, M. (1983). Ten whistleblowers and how they fared. *The Hastings Center Report, Dec.,* 33–41.

Kirk, R. (1986). The nurse executive as risk taker. *Journal of Nursing Administration, 16*(7), 9–12.

Lippitt, G. (1983). Courage: In common with a giraffe. *Training and Development Journal, Jan*, 89.

Means, P. (1989, Apr. 24–30). Would be whistle-blowers ought to first find a new job. *L.A. Business Journal*, pp. 11, 33.

Meyerowitz, S. A. (1985). Save your business from a wrongful discharge suit. *ABA Journal, 71*, 66–71.

Murphy, P. (1981). Deciding to blow the whistle. *American Journal of Nursing, Sept.*, 1692.

Nader, R., Petkas, P.J. & Blackwell, K. (Eds.). (1972). *Whistleblowing*. New York: Bantam Books.

O'Kane v. Board of Registered Nursing, 3 Civ. 19616, C.A. 3rd, Apr. 1, 1982.

O'Sullivan v. Mallon, 150 N.J. Super, 416, 390A.2d149 (1978).

Pierce v. Ortho Pharmaceutical Corp., 417 A 2d 505 (NJ1980).

Price, D. M. & Murphy, P. (1983). How and when to blow the whistle on unsafe practices. *Nursing Life, Jan./Feb.*, 52.

Reed, B. (1980). *The verdict.* New York: Simon & Schuster.

Regan, W. A. (1982). Intensive care nursing; doctor problems. *Regan Report on Nursing Law, Sept. 23*, 4.

Rookard v. Health and Hospitals Corp., No. 82-7739 (S.D.N.Y.1982).

Shank, B. (1959). Not now. In *Fragments* (p. 48). Englewood Cliffs, NJ: Prentice-Hall.

Smith, C. S. (1980). Outrageous or outraged: A nurse advocate story. *Nursing Outlook, Oct.*, 625.

Stecklow, S. (1988, Feb 18). Errors called widespread at Qiuffre. *The Philadelphia Inquirer*, p. 1.

Steinbock, B. (1983). The removal of Mr. Herbert's feeding tube. *The Hastings Center Report, Oct., 13–16.*

Stevens, A. (1988, Sept. 21). Nurse who challenged doctor's decision awarded $114,000 by jury. *Los Angeles Times.*

Tameny v. Atlantic Richfield Co. 610 P. 2d1330 (Calif. 1980).

Tobias, P. H. (1989). Can you help me? I've been fired. *ABA Journal, 70*, 68–71.

Toth v. Community Hospital at Glencove, 22.N.Y.2d255,292 N.Y.S.2d,239 N.E.2d,368(ct.App N.Y. 1968).

Trombettea v. Detroil, T.& I.R.R. Mich. APP. 489, 265 N.W.2d 385(1978).

Utter v. United Hospital Center, Inc. 236 S.E.2d213 (s.ct. West Va. 1977).

Witt, P. (1983). Notes of a whistleblower. *American Journal of Nursing, 83*, 1649–1651.

6

Institutional Forums

There have always been ethical issues in practice. Over the last 15 years technological, social, and economic changes have intensified the debate. Who should receive an intensive care unit bed? Who should receive an organ transplant? Should certain healthcare resources not be available to individuals when they reach a certain age? Should certain types of treatment only be available to those individuals who can pay for it? Doctors have at their disposal a vast array of interventions that, when combined with specific treatments, often unnecessarily prolong survival. People are living longer with serious chronic diseases, and money to pay for everything is getting very scarce.

The names of Quinlan, Barber, Bartling, and Brophy, to name just a few, have appeared in newspaper headlines across the country. These court cases challenged what healthcare professionals believed was the right thing to do. The language used to describe the dilemmas was new to most healthcare professionals. The principles that should guide decision making were unfamiliar, required different problem-solving skills, and necessitated the involvement of professionals outside the traditional healthcare community. Additionally, a different way to interact was needed for the professionals within the healthcare institution.

It was being recognized that effective institutional mechanisms were necessary to address the ethical issues arising in healthcare. The notion of having established forums for multidisciplinary deliberation has received considerable attention. Various professional publications, including nursing, medicine, and hospital administration journals, have discussed three different forums that can be operationalized in most healthcare settings: the institutional ethics committee, the nursing ethics council, and unit-based ethics rounds.

Institutional Ethics Committee

The concept of a committee to review ethical issues got an interesting beginning in the 1920s, reviewing sterilization requests. In the 1950s and 1960s hospitals formed abortion review committees. Prior to *Roe v. Wade* some states allowed abortion only if the pregnant woman's life was in danger (Levine, 1984). During the late 1960s patient selection committees were used to decide which of the candidates for kidney dialysis would receive the life-saving treatment. The Scribner shunt had been invented, but there were not enough dialysis machines to meet the growing demand. Dr. Scribner's affiliated hospital, University Hospital in Seattle, created a committee to decide who would get placed on dialysis. Those who did not get the machine died. Various patient criteria were used to make the decision. The fact that most recipients were male, married, employed, and between the ages of 25 and 45 contributed to the uneasiness in the country when these facts were made public (Beauchamp & Childress, 1983). Exposure of the committee's decisions paved the way for Medicare in 1972 to fund dialysis for all patients with end-stage renal disease. The controversy ended, and the committee's purpose became obsolete.

Institutional review boards (IRBs) designed to protect human research subjects have existed in most hospitals since the early 1970s. When Barney Clark received his artificial heart under the research protocol, a multidisciplinary committee reviewed his medical history and suitability prior to approving him as a candidate (Annas, 1983).

The concept of the institutional ethics committee (IEC) first came to public attention in the 1976 Karen Ann Quinlan case. The New Jersey Supreme Court proposed "prognosis committees" that could convene to deliberate an individual patient's prognosis (*In re Quinlan,* 1976). The court did not actually conceptualize a committee that would discuss broad ethical issues. Though interest in such committees did occur across the country, there was not widespread movement by hospitals to establish IECs. In 1983 the President's Commission for the Study of Ethical Problems in Medical and Biomedical Behavioral Research emphasized using informal procedures rather that formal ones such as the courts to review cases involving life or death issues (President's Commission for the Study of Ethical Problems in Medicine and Biomedical and Behavioral Research, 1983). It was not until the federal government issued the final Baby Doe regulations that committee formation intensified. The regulations called for the establishment of infant care review committees in hospitals caring for newborns (*Federal Register,* 1984). At that time, many hospitals initiated infant care review committees to demonstrate their willingness to monitor their own activities. Hospitals hoped that such voluntary mechanisms would be preferable to the use of hotlines to enforce what many believed to be unnecessary regulations.

In 1982 only 1% of hospitals had ethics committees (Younger, Jackson, Coulton, Juknialis, & Smith, 1983). A 1983 survey by the American Hospital Association's National Society of Patient Representatives reported that 26% of hospitals had a formal or informal group that functioned as an IEC ("Hospital Ethics Committees," 1984). Experts say the numbers continue to grow. A 1985 study reported that two-thirds of the hospitals surveyed (out of 200) had infant care review committees. A 1988 study of all hospitals belonging to the National Association of Children's Hospitals and Related Institutions (NACHRI) reported that 58 hospitals out of 87 had an institutional ethics committee (Levine-Ariff, 1988). A 1988 survey of all acute care hospital members of the Hospital Council of Southern California reported that 65% of the hospitals had ethics committees (American Hospital Association, 1988). In 1988, Maryland became the first state to require hospitals to form ethics committees. The concept of hospital ethics committees has been endorsed by the American Hospital Association, American Academy of Pediatrics, NACHRI, the American Nurses' Association, the Catholic Health Association, the American Medical Association, and the American College of Health Care Executives. In 1984 the American Hospital Association published general guidelines on establishment of hospital committees to consider biomedical ethical issues. As institutional ethics committees proliferate, discussions about optimal membership, functions, and authority have intensified.

Membership

The generic make-up or membership of the IEC is not universally agreed upon. However, as an ethics committee, it should represent what ethicists term the "community of moral discourse." Thus it should be reflective of the diversity of the healthcare community. That is to say, IECs should be mutlidisciplinary. They may include nurses and physicians, as well as social workers, experts in ethics, lawyers, hospital administrators, clergy, and community members. The representation of the committee will depend upon the nature and size of the institution. The presence of community members is an attempt to keep decisions from being strictly an in-house process. Clergy are often utilized in this capacity, as well as for their background in ethical decision making.

The inclusion of an attorney is not viewed as necessary by all committees. Their presence could bias the members toward a legal approach when making ethical decisions. An attorney who also represents the hospital could potentiate a conflict of interest. Certainly, legal concerns must be addressed, but such opinions can be sought without having an attorney on the committee. When a point of law is raised, attorneys are better utilized as consultants.

An ethicist sitting on the committee should be someone with a knowledge of healthcare. Otherwise, the committee members will continually find themselves explaining the hospital environment. Since there may be a tendency for other members to defer to the ethicist, this individual should act as a facilitator for the discussion.

The physician complement should be representative of the diversity of medical practice in the institution. For example, a community hospital might have an internist, an obstetrician, a pediatrician, a neurologist, and a surgeon. At a children's hospital, a pediatrician, a neonatologist, an intensivist, a neurologist, and a surgeon would not be considered excessive.

In turn, nursing membership could include an administrator, a nurse manager, a clinical nurse specialist, and a staff nurse. The latter three individuals should represent different nursing specialties.

Traditionally, nursing membership has been defined per medical specialty, that is, a nurse from the intensive care unit, from obstetrics, from pediatrics, and perhaps from a specialized program. Using these criteria may limit selection to individuals because of where they work, not interest, skill in group process, knowledge about ethical decision making, or an ability to view the issues from a broader perspective. Obviously, a combination of positions and clinical specialties could be used. The inclusion of a nursing administrator would facilitate a committee that may set institutional policies and/or guidelines. The nursing administrator could contribute the overall nursing department's perspective, and in many organizations, the nursing administrator could represent hospital administration.

Younger, in his 1982 study, reported that physicians accounted for 57% of the committee membership, with three committees being composed entirely of physicians and hospital administrators being represented more often than nurses. The study of children's hospitals reported that 71% of the committees had the same number of nurse and physician members. However, on the average, there were 1.36 nurses versus 2.6 physicians on the committees (Levine-Ariff, 1988).

The National Commission on Nursing, composed of nurses, physicians, and administrators, reported that a major issue for the nursing profession is relationships among the nursing department, the medical staff, and hospital administration, including the individual nurse's ability to participate in decision making as it relates to nursing (Secretary's Commission on Nursing, 1988). Institutional ethics committees recommend action in many areas that impinge directly or indirectly on nurses and nursing care. Nurses are frequently caught in the middle of ethical dilemmas involving disagreements over patient care, with no forum for explicit discussion and resolution of these dilemmas. Committees that select equal representation from nursing and medicine will facilitate face-to-face discussion about the ethical issues that concern both professions. They will support environments more conducive to bringing to the surface a variety of perspectives. Experience has demonstrated that this type of interaction facilitates communication and a better understanding between all of the professionals.

To ensure diversity and to be fair, the committee should be representative of the institutional community. It is most important that all committee members be individuals who can look beyond their own beliefs and view issues from the patient's perspective. The members should also have a desire to become informed about ethical theory and principles, as well as the current issues of the day. "But the most exquisitely representative committee will do no good if its members are not thoughtful, reflective, critical thinkers who are willing and able to move slowly, to tolerate substantial ambiguity, and to accept and respect one another" (Ross, Bayley, Michel, & Pugh, 1986).

Functions

Generally, IECs serve to provide education, formulate guidelines for decision making, and consult on individual cases. It is generally agreed that initially, IECs should educate themselves and only then embark on other activities. A 1988 study of children's hospitals demonstrated that 94% of the ethics committees provide consultation. Educational activities followed in frequency, with 45% of the committees providing this function. Only 23% of the committees developed guidelines for decision making (Levine-Ariff, 1988). Providing ethics education and developing guidelines will be discussed more fully later in this chapter.

Case Review

Individual case review is an important function of any committee. Ethics committees naturally tend to want to move quickly to the case review role, perhaps because it is closer to the action or more rewarding than the slow process of providing education or developing guidelines. It is our experience that it takes approximately 2 years for ethics committee members to feel comfortable with each other and to effectively consider the issues. "For an ethics committee to fill a case review function effectively, the members must have the capacity to care about the opinions of fellow members, be comfortable with their understanding of ethical thinking and analysis, and have a high degree of credibility within the hospital community (Ross et al., 1986).

Ethical issues are not scheduled in advance and do not occur only between the hours of 9 to 5, Monday through Friday. In order to be responsive, an IEC may need to develop a smaller group that can be convened quickly. To allow prompt consideration of urgent questions, some ethics committees may designate one person to respond, but this approach can lead to a bias in decision making toward the designated person's profession. A better solution is to form a smaller consultative group composed of several persons from the committee: a nurse, a physician, an ethicist, and perhaps a member from another discipline. This smaller group would review the medical prognosis, provide emotional support, facilitate communication, clarify legal questions, and apply ethical principles for decision making. They could meet with the patient and family to clarify facts. A multidisciplinary group will ensure that facts are gathered from a variety of caregivers. This minimizes potential distortions of the facts due to stress and/or personal bias.

A survey by Perkins and Saathoff (1988) found that 98% of physicians reported "learning much" from the consultation. Also, 32% of the consultations identified a previously unrecognized ethical issue, and there was a 93% increase in the physician's confidence in the clinical, ethical decision-making process. There is no similar study done on nurses known to the authors. However, experience supports similar conclusions.

Retrospective case review should be done in the larger consultative committee. A case where the outcome and/or process raised ethical concerns could be reviewed. This type of analysis allows for thoughtful discussion, provides an educational opportunity for the committee, and helps identify preventive measures for the future.

The IEC can provide a forum where ethical issues that arise in practice can be raised and discussed. As ethics committees respond to cases, personnel concerns, legal problems, and communication failures are likely to present themselves in the guise of ethical issues. Managers on the committee can be very helpful in facilitating the process and directing the issue to a particular individual or group within the institution for appropriate resolution.

It is the nature of ethical issues that not every issue brought to the committee will reach resolution. A case brought to the ethics committee that points up the problems with allocation of intensive care beds may require much more discussion and input from others within the organization. This type of issue may contribute to the development of "preventive ethics" as guidelines are developed for the allocation of intensive care unit beds when census is high.

Access

Access to the committee should be available to any physician, health care employee, patient, or family member. An IEC that limits access to any one particular group (i.e., physicians) will not be able to effectively resolve many issues that are occurring at the bedside. It will certainly not facilitate a concern for patients' interest over those of the healthcare professional.

The committee should develop a procedure to make access easy for any individual who may need a consultation. Some ethics committees have developed specific brochures to explain their purpose and availability. Written information of this type can be provided to hospital staff. Some hospitals give these pamphlets to patients and families upon admission.

Organization

There are several options for where the committee is placed in the organization. It can be a committee of the medical staff, an administrative committee, or it can be a committee of the board of trustees. The latter is less common but is gaining in recognition because of the broad institutional impact of many of the committees' recommendations. A 1988 study of children's hospitals reported that 55% of their committees were under the medical staff, 32% were under hospital administration, and 7% were under the board of directors (Levine-Ariff, 1988).

The organizational structure of such committees may depend on concerns about discoverability of the proceedings. State laws differ on the issue. Many states provide immunity for records of certain medical staff committees whose function it is to review the quality of patient care. As a committee of the medical staff, the chairperson is usually a physician. However, some ethics committees have appointed co-chairpersons, with one of the individuals being a nonphysician.

Authority

There are several models for IEC authority. Mandatory-mandatory requires the hospital staff and/or physicians to submit specific types of cases for review and then requires that the recommendations of the IEC be mandatory. This model is the least common in practice. The mandatory-optional model requires review of certain cases, but the recommendations are optional. The optional-optional model requires no specific case review, and the recommendations are, again, optional. The last type of committee structure is the one most often utilized. However, some beginning committees may ask that certain cases come to the committee prospectively. For example, the impetus for the formation of the committee may have been concerns about how decisions to withhold and/or withdraw life-sustaining treatment were being made. While it is possible for an IEC to function in an actual decision making capacity, most authorities believe they function best in an advisory capacity. Ultimate decision making should remain at the bedside.

Documentation

Should an ethics committee document its consultation? If the consultation is not entered into the patient's record, where is the accountability for the professionals making recommendations? Where will such findings be recorded for future reference? Many committees are grappling with this. The legal implications for the institution have not been well established.

Frequency of Committee Meetings

The establishment of a formal committee, as opposed to an ad hoc group, fosters a group process that allows for some agreement on the principles that guide decision making. It allows time for the members of the group to develop a working relationship, which is critical for this type of committee. Regular meetings provide time to discuss issues prospectively as well as concurrently. In the children's hospitals study, 43% of the committees reported having meetings once a month; 3% meet twice a month; 19% meet every other month; and 29% only convene upon request (Levine-Ariff, 1988). The differences in activities and group process can only be speculated upon. No specific questions in the survey addressed this area.

Advantages and Disadvantages

The concept of the IEC continues to be a much-debated subject. Some of the possible disadvantages include:

- Infringement on the responsibility of professionals
- Infringement on the family's role
- Domination by one profession or ideology
- Diffusion of responsibility for decision making
- Acting as the institution's advocate, rather than the patient's

Though these are valid concerns, they can be avoided. Broadening the membership, especially the smaller consultative group, should minimize domination by one profession or ideology. Affirming the principle of autonomy and understanding the role of surrogate decision makers should facilitate decision making by the appropriate individual. Thus the committee should be able to keep a clear focus on the patient and not exclusively on the institution. Making recommendations and acting as a consultant, rather than as a decision maker, should minimize the committee's "interference" in the professionals' role. Finally, IECs have actually aided decision making by patients or families by minimizing paternalistic attitudes.

Advantages of an IEC include

- Providing a forum for communication
- Providing support to staff and families
- Preventing or minimizing ethical issues
- Potentially minimizing legal risk
- Allowing for some agreement on the principles that should guide decision making

Although these advantages may look like functions, they are not the reasons that IECs are established. They are an outgrowth of such a group process.

The current literature is supportive of institutional ethics committees. "The strength of ethics committees is their availability as a forum and whatever persuasive force each commands. At the same time, the limitations of committees are real; not all committees are equally strong" (Wolf, 1986). Hospitals that have a well-organized and functional review committee are in a better position to address difficult ethical dilemmas than those that do not. By keeping up to date on the legal and legislative changes that may impact ethical decision making, ethics committees can be a valuable resource for current thinking on an issue. Although the courts and federal regulations have stimulated the creation of institutional ethics committees, their development has filled a much-needed void in healthcare decision making. "A committee mechanism generally assumes that collaboration and rational analysis are likely to yield better decisions than those formulated by individuals alone or without critical reflection" (Kliegman, Mahowald, & Younger, 1986). Obviously, there are many times when ethical issues are adequately addressed by patients, families, and the caregivers. However, sometimes the complexity of decision making, coupled with obvious disagreement about what the outcome should be and/or who should decide, invites ethics committee consultation.

Committee Quality Assurance

Finally, each ethics committee must establish a periodic review process for the committee's functions and activities. They must ask themselves questions such as these: How well did the committee resolve differences of opinion? Were all sides of the issue presented? Did the committee members treat each other as shared decision makers? Did health care professionals believe they gained information or perspective about the dilemma? Were ethical principles highlighted during the discussion? Did legal opinions influence decision making? Were recommendations related to the best interest of the patient? Were autonomous patients given informed choice? Has the committee developed measures to prevent or at least minimize recurring ethical issues? "We must always examine what we have done, either to decide that it was right and continue or to decide that it was wrong and change (Bason, 1984). Institutional ethics committees cannot be viewed as a quick fix for bioethical dilemmas in the institutional setting. They are but one tool for promoting both individual and institutional sensitivity about bioethics. A forum where ethical dilemmas can be raised should reduce the influence of misinformation, individual bias, and misguided good will.

Nursing Ethics Council

Another mechanism that can be developed within a healthcare institution is a nursing ethics council, in addition to or in conjunction with an IEC. Nurses and physicians alike often question why nurses need their own ethics committee.

Nursing ethics is clearly distinct from medical ethics. The issues nurses face at the bedside are different from those of physicians. "Many conflicts arise from the nurse's complex role, so that they can be grouped under the heading of the 'nurse in the middle' problem. The nurse often appears to be in the position of having great responsibilities, required to have many skills, and yet in possession of few decision powers" (Jameton, 1977). Nurses also have a different perspective about many of the issues that arise in practice. For a nurse, talking with a dying patient is not simply knowing what to tell. A nurse listens for a patient's understanding of his/her prognosis, a decision to pursue or not pursue recommended treatment, a desire to die at home, a need to have all medical treatment stopped, a need for pain medication, and so on. The nurse discusses these concerns with patients and helps them to achieve their wishes.

Ethical issues specific to nurses themselves rarely get discussed at an IEC. The nurse's role in informed consent or issues involving impaired nurses, nurse staffing ratios, the allocation of nursing resources, or a nurse's refusal of assignment are but a few examples. Ethical issues create questions about a nurse's role and her relationships with other professionals. "Much medical ethics discussion proceeds on the simplifying assumption that one professional is making decisions. Although this fiction may work as a representation of medical decision-making, any work on ethics in nursing must recognize a multiplicity of professional agents" (Jameton, 1977).

Objectives of a nursing ethics council might include

- To educate nurses in ethical theory and principles
- To educate the nursing staff in the differences between nursing and medical ethical dilemmas
- To educate nurses about the Code for Nurses and its application to practice
- To serve as a resource to address and clarify nursing ethical issues
- To provide resource material (e.g., journal articles and audiovisuals)
- To discuss and clarify current ethical issues
- To provide input into the hospital IEC

The council can also serve as a sounding board before taking an issue to the IEC. One of the primary functions of the nursing council, like the IEC, is education. Too often, nurses do not clearly identify issues as ethical ones or have difficulty describing their concerns. They lack the language and theory to communicate their moral concerns in a specific and convincing manner. Thus they respond emotionally or report that something "just isn't right." A nursing council can provide ongoing opportunities for nurses to refine their ability to articulate the issues more clearly and incorporate ethical principles into clinical practice.

It is important for the nursing ethics council to be facilitated by a nurse. Discussions that focus on nursing practice can best be led by a nurse who is familiar with the values of the nursing profession. Ideally, this nurse would be a nurse ethicist or a nurse educated in ethical theory and its application to clinical practice.

The nursing ethics council should develop a format for case discussion separate from the medical model of case presentation. The example shown in Chapter 3, "Ethical Decision Making," is one such format. As was explained in that chapter, the model can be used as a guide to elicit appropriate information and does not have to be used in a structured format. Consistency with one mode of presentation will reinforce the ethics perspective of the case and increase the participants' comfort level. Unless alternative modes of analysis are provided, it is easy to lapse into a discussion about electrolyte imbalances and psychosocial aberrations, as examples.

Additionally, nurses should have some idea of what to expect when they call a member of the nursing committee for consultation. A nurse unfamiliar with ethical decision making would be helped by the council members. Questions would be asked to elicit needed information before recommendations are given. Figure 6.1 is an example of information that can be provided to each nurse on the staff. It outlines the procedure to bring a concern to the council and the general format for discussion.

A nursing ethics council works best when it is comprised of interested members, rather than appointed representatives. Ideally, the nursing committee should be representative of the diversity of nursing

NURSING ETHICS COMMITTEE CASE PRESENTATION

1. Dilemma is brought to attention of ethics committee member.
2. Member contacts Chairperson of ethics committee and explains the issue.
3. The Chairperson, together with the member, decides whether issues are urgent or if can wait until the next meeting.
4. Urgent issues are discussed on the nursing unit. Committee members and staff that can be present gather to discuss case.
5. Nurse (presenter) is allotted 10 minutes in which to present the issues. The nurse may include any team members he/she feels may add to the presentation.
6. Discussion occurs, ethical issue(s) clarified, questions and answers from members occur.
7. Recommendations given.

Figure 6.1. Nursing ethics committee case presentations.

roles in the organization: a staff nurse, clinical nurse specialist, nurse practitioner, nurse manager, and nurse administrator might all be represented on the council. Many nurses in the different clinical specialty areas consider their ethical issues to be unique, so all clinical specialties should be represented. However, it is surprising how many issues are similar. Resource utilization, informed consent, withholding and withdrawal of treatment, and the use of technology are but a few examples of common ground. The differences lie in the frequency of a particular issue, the intensity and variety of clinical concerns that form the backdrop for the dilemma, and the level of collaboration between the nurse and the doctor. This does not mean to imply that there are no differences. In fact, certain clinical areas may want to have specific attention paid to their specialty. The field of obstetrics, as an example, raises questions of the innocent third party and the rights of the pregnant woman that are very specific to the specialty. The intensive care unit brings to mind specific questions about withdrawal of life-sustaining treatment and the responsibilities of the nurse. The pediatric area raises very specific concerns about informed consent for minors. The oncology service raises issues about treatment options versus patients' wishes to die at home. Having various groups of nurses listen to others' particular dilemmas brings objectivity and a broad perspective to decision making. Sometimes discussion of these concerns can be best accomplished by using ethics rounds, which will be explored in the next section.

Case Examples

Consider these cases that could come to a nursing ethics committee:

- An 8-year-old child with cystic fibrosis, well known to the hospital, was admitted in severe respiratory distress. Within 2 days, the child's condition worsened, and it was felt that he would not survive this hospitalization. The child's parents were dead. He was being raised by his sister, who had a poor history of compliance with medical treatments. The sister was approached for a Do Not Resuscitate order, but she refused. She wanted everything done. Two days later, the child's condition deteriorated. The sister was called but could not be reached. The physician believed that he had to intubate the child. The child was placed on a ventilator and died the next day.

  Two weeks after the incident, the nurse involved presented the case to the nursing ethics council. She stated that she could not shake the vision of the child being intubated and wanted to know if there was something else she should have done. Various committee members shared similar situations and related what they had done. The group leader directed the discussion to the options. The nurse clearly believed that the patient was being harmed and yet felt helpless to prevent the intubation. The options discussed were be firm when speaking with the physician and state your objections in ethical terms; say that "if this intervention occurs, I cannot continue to deliver care"; physically block the physician; immediately get some other clinical support and or managerial support. These options were not stated in preferential order. The various options were discussed as well as the risks involved with each one. Additionally, there was discussion about prospectively speaking with the child and sister. Upon leaving the committee, the nurse felt better about what she did do but still felt angry and frustrated about the outcome. The nursing ethics committee provided a forum for the nurse to raise concerns particular to the nursing profession. More important, it gave the nurse an opportunity to do something different the next time.

- A 25-year-old patient with hemophilia and AIDS was admitted to the hospital in a debilitated state. He was still alert, but there were signs of progressive central nervous system deterioration. The patient had a wife and no children. The patient had begun to talk with the nurse about dying. The primary nurse shared this information with the physician and encouraged truthfulness about prognosis and discussion about potential withholding or withdrawal of treatments. The physician stated that the patient was a fighter, and he wasn't giving up on him. The nurse pursued this line of communication with one of the patient's consulting physicians. Neither physician talked with the patient about the realities of his prognosis. The patient continued to speak to the nurse about his concern for the future. The nurse came to the nursing ethics council to clarify the options and for help to explain her concerns in ethical terms. The ethics council explained the ethical concepts and suggested various options: Help the patient talk with the physician, call a multidisciplinary case conference to discuss the issues, call a case conference with the family, and/or take the case to the hospital IEC. The committee helped the nurse enumerate the questions to which clear answers had not been given: What was the prognosis? What did the patient want? How involved was the wife? These were but a few. The nurse was then able to help the patient communicate to the entire healthcare team. This particular nurse left the committee feeling as if she could act positively as a patient advocate.

The nursing committee, as a whole, may want to take a position on certain nursing concerns, either those that affect all nurses or those within a particular specialty. For example, the nurse's role in organ transplantation, obtaining informed consent, or withdrawing life-sustaining treatment could be considered as potential statements. But the ethics council must recognize that they are part of a larger community. Their education of all nursing staff will facilitate consensus on certain issues, which may be documented in a departmental philosophy, policy, or standards for practice. Additionally, a nursing ethics council that has a strong voice on the IEC and works closely with that committee in the formation of its policies or guidelines may be able to incorporate nursing's specific concerns within a multidisciplinary position statement. Each organization must decide how best to proceed. The important point is that nursing concerns must not take a back seat to the wishes of other professionals or the institution.

Initially, the formation of a nursing council takes the commitment of just a few people. Resources, both informational and human, should be identified. Literature, such as the documents, books, and articles identified at the end of this is a good place to begin. Contacting colleges of nursing, state nursing associations, and local college and university philosophy departments may help identify individuals skilled in bioethical issues. The American Nurses' Association and some state nurses' associations have ethics committees. The American Association of Critical-Care Nurses also has a national ethics committee. These organizations can provide a wealth of resources. Contacting local hospitals, particularly teaching hospitals, may reveal the existence of a nursing ethics council.

Nursing ethics councils are a visible affirmation of nursing departmental support for a nurse's involvement in ethical decision making. A forum such as this can serve to strengthen nurse-to-nurse relationships and minimize the differences. The mere presence of the council will provide a valuable resource in facilitating positive outcomes for difficult situations.

Ethics Rounds

A third mechanism, employed either alone or in conjunction with an IEC or nursing ethics council, would be a regular pattern of ethics rounds.

Ethics rounds are similar to other rounds, in that participants discuss a case study in some organized fashion. In ethics rounds, the clinical aspects of the case become the backdrop for an organized discussion of the ethical dilemma and possible solutions. A brief medical and nursing history should be given, emphasizing specific facts relevant to the moral question(s). "To be helpful, these rounds must be regularly scheduled and carefully organized for fruitful discussions that do not disintegrate into grip sessions and rhetoric (Levine-Ariff, 1988). Organized ethics rounds require a skilled leader who serves as a group facilitator. This person's group leadership skills and knowledge of bioethical theories and principles are important factors in helping the group maintain a constructive focus. The group leader assists the participants in coming to terms with the ethical principles, patient/family preferences, and the available alternatives.

Ethics rounds can be multidisciplinary or confined to a homogeneous group, such as the nurses on one nursing unit. A multidisciplinary group could help facilitate communication between nurses and physicians. In general, both groups start with little knowledge about bioethics and do share some common values. If this is not possible, then nurses should meet alone or with other nonphysician disciplines. Ethics rounds can help the nurses become more confident and assertive in articulating their views, both in day-to-day situations and also on the occasion when they may present a case to the IEC.

Ethics rounds can discuss current or retrospective cases. If a current case is being discussed, it can be more effective to raise the issues early in the patient's hospital course. The potential then exists to offer a preventive approach to solving ethical concerns, instead of having decisions take place in a crisis milieu. The goal of these rounds is not to make clinical decisions but to discuss moral problems confronted by caregivers. Some objectives might be

- To develop the participants' skills in ethical decision making
- To increase awareness of the complexity of ethical decision making within a clinical context
- To promote discussion of all options in a given ethical dilemma
- To provide an environment where various professional attitudes and values are explored
- To enhance the caregivers' ability to identify moral issues

During ethics rounds, the discussion leader should engage in a great deal of give and take with the participants. Inconsistencies in reasoning can be pointed out, as well as alternatives to actions and unforeseen consequences of various decisions. Participants should feel free to share thoughts and opinions. Ethics rounds should promote open discussion and reflection rather than purposefully making recommendations about a particular issue.

The rounds can take place at the bedside or in a conference room. Participants should feel comfortable that the environment will not restrict discussion because of the presence of families or other groups unfamiliar with the format and confidential nature of the case. Reasonable time should be allocated for discussion, with the group leader keeping to the time constraints.

Ethics, in the context of clinical decision-making, identifies, analyzes, and attempts to resolve the moral problems that arise in patient care. The goal of a formal ethical decision making process is to foster a climate of quality patient care that is congruent with clear ethical standards. In the past, what was right and good for the patient was seen in relationship to the technical decisions made by the physician. Murphy (1984) writes that "the notion of ethics committees and shared health care decision making challenge (sic) the tradition of physicians as lone decision makers. It changes a perception that health care decisions are equated with medical decisions." Times have indeed changed. Ethical decisions still must take into account the recommendations of the physician but must also weigh more heavily the individual patient's values and preferences. Regular ethics rounds will foster an awareness of ethical principles and concepts in daily practice.

Ethics Education

All of the institutional mechanisms to aid decision making emphasize education as a primary objective. Ethics education helps practitioners make moral choices based on knowledge, rather than personal values and vague intuitions. In a 1977 survey, Aroskar found that only 7% of accredited BSN programs require course work in ethics or medical ethics. A recent report of the American Association of Colleges of Nursing reports a significant prevalence of ethics content in undergraduate nursing programs (Redmon & Cassells, 1988). Medical undergraduate programs relate the same trend (Bernard, 1988; Veatch & Sollitoo, 1976). Yet the majority of nurses practicing currently have probably not had the benefit of any ethics education. For those who have had formal education, applying ethical theory in situations where practitioners must bear the responsibility for their actions is a different matter.

Mayberry (1986) states that moral judgment tends to plateau when formal education is discontinued. Recognizing this fact and knowing that ethics education in the clinical setting helps health care practitioners make anticipatory decisions and gain confidence to carry out decisions it becomes incumbent upon management and ethics committees to incorporate ethics education into ongoing institutional education programs. In a published study of 1023 physicians' perceptions of how useful and relevant courses in medical ethics were to their practices, most thought these courses were valuable in their daily practice (Pellegrino et al., 1985). The American College of Healthcare Executives endorsed the development of defined programs and courses for ethics in undergraduate and graduate programs in healthcare administration, as well as in continuing education programs (Pirovano, 1986). Ethics education can be useful in providing guidance concerning the appropriate process of ethical decision making and increasing one's understanding about the principals that guide human behavior. It can help healthcare professionals approach ethical decisions with a firm background and knowledge of the issues.

Separating medical treatment decisions from moral questions facilitates communication. The study of ethics gives all healthcare practitioners a language to articulate their concerns. A common framework from which to speak facilitates mutual support across disciplines. The issues lose their emotional context, and it is easier for colleagues to understand and support an individual, thus it is easier to act ethically.

Implementing nurse-physician networking sessions is an example of how to accomplish a collaborative approach to ethics education between both nurses and physicians and staff and management. The forum is usually held in the evening, accompanied by food and socializing. It can be sponsored by the IEC or nursing and/or medical administration. Nurse and physician guests can present a short discussion about the benefits of IECs and the differences between nursing and medical ethics. A film, like *Code Gray* (Achtenberg, 1983), can help stimulate discussion. Where this technique has been used, it has been received positively. Usually, this type of ethics discussion is but one forum within the year's program.

By initiating educational opportunities, the nurse manager indicates that such issues are open to discussion and are an important part of nursing practice, thus making it possible for the staff to risk raising an issue. Nurses, physicians, philosophers, and others with a background and understanding about ethical decision making should be asked to provide the education.

Summary

Unfortunately, ethics education alone will not clear up the problems.

It will increase a nurse's ability to discuss the issues and reach toward a resolution. However, individual nurses who would usually act morally might not do so, simply because they are unaware of the ethical problems that lie hidden in situations they confront. Others will not discover a moral problem because they are so involved with the situation. Information on ethical theory and ethical decision making form the foundation from which to discuss the current issues of the day. Open discussion will raise the questions from which to explore the issues. Practicing within an ethical environment will facilitate the positive outcomes.

Patients must be confident that the decision making process takes into account the forces in society and the expectations they have about the health professionals who render care. It is a historical relationship based on trust. In order to honor that trust, health professionals faced with these issues need guidance from well-founded ethical principles and an environment that will support their implementation. An IEC, a nursing ethics council, and ethics education can support this endeavor.

REFERENCES

Achtenberg, B., Sawyer, J., & Mitchell, C. (1983). Code gray: Ethical dilemmas in nursing [Film]. Boston: Boston Film/Video Production.

American Hospital Association. (1984). *Guidelines: Hospital committees on biomedical ethics*. Chicago: Author.

American Hospital Association, Hospital Council of Southern California. (1988). Unpublished research.

Annas, G. J. (1983). The lion and the crocodiles: Consent to the artificial heart. *Hastings Center Report, 13,* 20–22.

Aroskar, M. A. (1977). Ethics in the nursing curriculum. *Nursing Outlook, 25,*260–264.

Bason, M. D. (1984). Bioethics in the medical center: An exploration. *Hospital Practice, 19*(7), 177–201.

Beauchamp, T. L., & Childress, J. F. (1983). *Principles of bioethics,* (2nd ed; p. 206). New York: Oxford University Press.

Bernard, D. (1988). Residency ethics teaching. *Archives of Internal Medicine, 148,*1836–1838.

Fast, N., Charley, C. (1986). What can a hospital ethics committee do for you? *Contemporary Pediatrics, Feb.,* 119.

Federal Register. (1984). Jan. 12., 49:1622–1654. Washington, DC: U.S. Government Printing Office.

Hospital ethics committees surveyed. (1984). *Hospitals, 58,* 52.

In re Quinlan: 70 N.J. 10, 355A, 2d647, 1976.

Jameton, A. (1977). The nurse: When roles and rules conflict. *Hastings Center Report, 7,* 22–23.

Kliegman, R. M., Mahowald, M. B., & Younger, S. J. (1986). In our best interests:

Experiences and workings of an ethics review committee. *Journal of Pediatrics, 108,* 2.

Levine, C. (1984). Questions and some very tentative answers about hospital ethics committees. *Hastings Center Report, 14,* 3, 9–12.

Levine-Ariff, J. (1988). Ethical forums. In *Nursing yearbook* (p. 209). Springhouse, PA: Springhouse.

Levine-Ariff, J. (1988). *Ethics committees in childrens' hospitals.* Unpublished research.

Mayberry, M.A. (1986). Ethical decision-making: a response of hospital nurses. *Nursing Administrative Quarterly, 10*(3), 75–81.

Murphy, C.P. (1984). The changing role of nurses in making ethical decisions. *Law, Medicine, & Healthcare, 12,* 173.

Pellegrino, E. D., Hart, R. J., Henderson, S. R., et al. (1985). Relevance and usefulness of courses in medial ethics: A survey of physicians' perspectives. *Journal of the American Medical Association, 253,* 49–53.

Perkins, H., Saathoff, B. (1988). Impact of medical ethics consultation on physicians: An exploratory study. *American Journal of Medicine,* Dec. 85., 761–763.

Pirovano, D. O. (1986). *The buck stops on health care ethics? Coordinator, Feb.,*28–29.

President's Commission for the Study of Ethical Problems in Medicine and Biomedical and Behavioral Research. (1983). Deciding to forego life-sustaining treatment. Washington, DC: Government Printing Office.

Redman, B. K., Cassells, J. M. (1988). The ethical education of the RN. *The Hastings Center Report, 18,* 2–30.

Ross, J. W., Bayley, S. C., Michel, V., & Pugh, D. (1986). *Handbook for hospital ethics committees.* Chicago: American Hospital Association.

Secretary's Commission on Nursing. (1988). *Final report.* Washington, DC: Department of Health and Human Services.

Veatch, R. M., & Sollitto, S. (1976). Medical ethics teaching. Report of a national medical school survey. *Journal of the American Medical Association, 235,* 1030–1033.

Wolf, Susan M. (1986). Ethics committees in the courts. *The Hastings Center Report, 16,* 12–16.

Younger, S. J., Jackson, D. L., Coulton, C., Juknialis, B. W., & Smith, E. (1983). A national survey of hospital ethics committees. In President's Commission for the Study of Ethical Problems in Medicine and Biomedical and Behavioral Research, *Deciding to Forego Life-Sustaining Treatment.* Washington, DC: Government Printing Office.

7

Ethical Guidelines

Jameton's statement about moral distress is particularly relevant to any understanding of why organizations and professional associations may want to implement guidelines or position statements. "Moral distress arises when one knows the right thing to do, but institutional constraints make it nearly impossible to pursue the right course of action" (Jameton, 1984). Outdated policies, nonexistent ones, a resistive hierarchy, an environment that limits discussion of ethical issues, or uncertainty about what is the right thing to do necessitate the need for current guidelines and position statements. Position statements developed by professional associations can provide guidance to healthcare practitioners struggling to balance professional duties and organizational demands. Institutional guidelines can provide a framework to structure decision making and to ensure consideration of the relevant facts and values. Both can help to reassure society that these important decisions are made with careful deliberation and accountability.

Position Statements

Position statements are usually written by professional associations. They are general statements that delineate the important concepts inherent in a particular ethical issue. They often clarify moral uncertainty. "Moral uncertainty arises when one is unsure what moral principles or values apply, or even what the moral problem is" (Jameton, 1984). But perhaps more importantly, they establish normative standards for the "values, obligations, and ideals of the professions they represent" (Fowler, 1988).

The American Nurses' Association Committee on Ethics has completed various position statements on issues such as withholding or withdrawing food and fluid. The American Association of Critical-Care Nurses Ethics Committee has published a position statement on advocacy. Various state nurses' associations have also been involved in developing position statements on various ethical issues. The California Nurses' Association has published a position statement on withholding and withdrawing treatment. The Massachusetts Nurses' Association has prepared a statement on patient protection. Copies of these statements are available from the different associations.

Through these position statements, these professional associations are giving attention to the moral concerns of nurses. These documents are crucial for the practice of nursing. They set standards for ethical practice and provide a substantial resource to which the nurse can turn for support and guidance. They give notice and attention to nursing's particular ethical concerns.

Institutional Guidelines

The particular contribution of guidelines lies with helping healthcare professionals prospectively plan for ethical issues that require prompt intervention, such as requests from families to withdraw food and fluids. Guidelines provide an opportunity to discuss how future cases should be handled. Sometimes, without guidance as to the approach the healthcare team should take, increased suffering for patients, families, and the involved professionals may occur. It is certainly true, though, that if poorly designed or wrongly applied, decision making protocols can legitimize bad decisions, diffuse responsibility, or be too rigid. Institutional guidelines are not a panacea, nor do they make final decisions easier. However, thoughtfully designed guidelines are a feasible method to foster clinical decisions that are responsive to both the needs of patients and the obligations of institutions and professionals.

Any discussion about setting institutional guidelines to aid decision making would be incomplete without focusing on their content and development within the organization.

First, the committee must determine what particular issues have caused concerns. The committee should be aware of frequent situations that have led to problems with withholding and withdrawing life-sustaining treatment, as one example. If specific concerns arise infrequently, they may not warrant a policy. However, a single situation may have caused such extreme turmoil, and even though it may occur only occasionally, a policy may be warranted. Generally, institutional guidelines or policies should reflect current thinking in the field of ethical decision making. The committee may find it helpful to gather policies from other hospitals. A particular hospital's policy should not be accepted blindly. The committee owes the other healthcare practitioners, and in particular the patients, careful deliberation over the content of any policy it adopts. It can provide guidance to all concerned in areas such as withholding and withdrawing treatment, Do Not Resuscitate orders, and informed consent. They can provide an approach to decision making in general or relate specific content peculiar to individual treatment modalities. "Generally, they should cover 'macro' policy issues that transcend the treatment of any one person as well as 'micro' issues raised by the treatment of individual patients" (Smith & Veatch, 1987). They must consider not only patients with decision making capacity but also those without it. The guidelines should represent the broad healthcare team, emphasizing the unique roles of nurses and doctors. They must promote clinical practices that conform to public policies, including statutes, regulations, and common law, as well as reflecting voluntary standards. Voluntary standards may include JCAHO recommendations, as well as various healthcare professionals' codes of ethics and standards of practice.

Available data on the prevalence of decision making policies or guidelines are incomplete, although the data reveal a growth in the prevalence of such protocols. A 1986 study done by JCAHO reported on data obtained from a national survey (Longo, Warren, Roberts, & Dunlop, 1988). Four kinds of healthcare institutions were surveyed: acute care hospitals, long-term care facilities, psychiatric hospitals, and hospice organizations. Of the four types of institutions surveyed, acute care hospitals were the most likely to have a policy regarding resuscitation. Do Not Resuscitate policies were most common in large urban hospitals, especially those with academic or religious affiliation. Only 20% of all responding hospitals reported that they addressed issues of withholding and withdrawing treatments other than resuscitation. The fact that large numbers of hospitals have no decision making protocols, or only have ones that deal with resuscitation, increases the probability that treatment preferences would be carried out by chance, dependent on an individual practitioner's belief and not necessarily the wishes of patients and/or families. Effective January 1, 1988, the JCAHO required hospitals to establish formal DNR policies (Joint Commission on Accreditation of Healthcare Organizations, 1987).

Reflect on these situations:

Marge Lewis is a 55-year-old woman who has recently been diagnosed with inoperable abdominal cancer. She has been an active woman all of her life and remains in an alert state. She is asking the nurse questions about the results of her surgery. She had been told before surgery, by her physician, that her chances for recovery were very good. Her husband and doctor have told the nurse that they do not want Mrs. Lewis to know the truth, as she would just get severely depressed.

Baby girl Jones has been born with a hypoplastic left heart. She also has only one kidney and no spleen. She is deteriorating rapidly. Her parents, who love her desperately, want the suffering to end. They have requested that all treatment be stopped and the ventilator be withdrawn.

Ira Stern had lived a long, full life when, at the age of 50, he was diagnosed with ALS. He was having trouble breathing, and his wife brought him into the hospital in a near-unconscious state. He was immediately intubated and admitted to the intensive care unit. In the emergency room, a nurse believed Mr. Stern had resisted the intubation and subsequent interventions. The wife was questioned as to her husband's wishes for such treatment. Mrs. Stern said they wanted everything done. After admission to the intensive care unit, the patient's private physician arrived. He discussed with the nursing staff the patient's previous clear expressions to him about treatment choice. The physician stated that Mr. Stern did not want to be placed on a ventilator, knowing that he would never come off. The nursing staff relayed Mrs. Stern's comments.

Institutional guidelines improve clinical decision making. They will decrease staff's uncertainties about what practices are permitted, who gets to decide, and what are the obligations of healthcare professionals. Guidelines reduce arbitrary decision making and improve accountability for those decisions. They should affirm patient autonomy and truth telling as important principles. They would support Marge Lewis's right to know, within an environment that reflects Mr. Lewis's feelings and concerns.

Through guidelines, organizational means would be set forth to honor patients' requests before greater harm is done. There would be recognition that decisions to treat are not irrevocable, and prospective treatment plans would be created so that Mr. Stern could have his wishes honored without additional suffering. Protocols would recognize a parent's right to make treatment decisions for his/her child, emphasizing professional intervention only when it was absolutely felt that the parents were not acting in the best interests of their child.

Appropriate procedures would clarify how the healthcare professional and institution should proceed under such circumstances.

Patients have a right to fully understand an institution's position on major moral issues such as withholding and withdrawing life support treatments, withdrawal of food and fluids, resuscitation, abortion, and the care of dying patients. In some communities, the availability of more than one institution would allow patients to choose hospitals whose beliefs are compatible with their own.

In 1987 the New Jersey Supreme Court would not support a nursing home's wish to discharge a patient whose desire to have food and fluids withdrawn was morally objectional to the facility (*In re Jobes,* 1986). The court ordered the nursing home to discontinue the tube feedings for Nancy Jobes, who was in a persistent vegetative state. The court stated that the nursing home's policy against withholding nutritional support was unwritten and the patient's family had never been informed of such a policy (*In re Jobes,* 1987).

At the same time, we must recognize that institutions are made up of individuals who have their own beliefs and values. The value that society places on individual freedoms and voluntarism weighs against compelling healthcare practitioners to carry out treatment decisions to which they object. The Code for Nurses affirms a nurse's right to refuse to participate in specific treatment situations. However, it is incumbent upon the nurse not to abandon the patient. The nurse must find another nurse of equal competence to care for the patient. An orderly transfer of the patient to the care of others should occur. Organizations must develop protocols that address this critical area. For example, in a situation where it is in a patient's best interest to have food and fluids withdrawn, some nurses may find it difficult to take care of this patient on a frequent basis, other nurses may not want to care for this patient at all, and yet some other nurses, who may have established a relationship with the patient and family, may want to render care whenever they are on duty.

The nurse manager must provide an environment where these concerns can be openly raised and the nurses' wishes honored. The situation should then be thoroughly evaluated and group discussion occur, so the manager can become clear about the staff's concerns. Situations of this nature may involve major objections to the clinical decisions. Sometimes it is simply a lack of information that has prompted nursing's objections. At times, the nurse manager may need to call an immediate multidisciplinary case conference to help resolve issues. Nurse managers can support individual nurses at case conferences where these issues may be discussed. The nurse manager can be present or ensure the presence of other nurses adept at articulating the issues. Policies focusing on dispute resolution would serve both the staff and management.

Clearly, the development of guidelines requires an organization that has both knowledge and motivation. Barriers to the development and implementation of protocols for ethical decision making range from private concerns about institutional interference in the practice of medicine to practical questions about who should be involved and how any written document can address succinctly all the variables. The latter concerns are perhaps the easiest to address first. An institutional ethics committee would be the obvious group to develop such protocols. Otherwise, the bringing together of a similar group of individuals would be reasonable. Outside input from ethicists or doctors and nurses well versed in ethical issues could be obtained. Yet it must be recognized that the development of decision making protocols occurs best as consensus builds. It may not be possible to initially achieve all desired ends.

Many healthcare professionals are not fully informed as to their institutional duties. They confuse ethical duties and legal duties. The latter are sometimes exaggerated by institutional attorneys or insurance companies who may not be well versed in recent developments in bioethics and may give inaccurate or unrealistic advice. They may state their opinions so emphatically that the health professional or institution may believe that the advice must be followed. Health professionals themselves may have difficulty discussing with families treatment options that include withholding or withdrawing treatment. Failure to cure weighs heavy on a physician who has not dealt with his own personal fear of failure. The physician who has not yet recognized that not curing is not necessarily related to failure may have a difficult time with guidelines that honor patient autonomy. Nurses and doctors often lack the words that could appropriately relay the issues, make recommendations, and reflect care and concern for individuals. Discussion and education over time may help facilitate communication. Meanwhile, those who can facilitate dialogue with patients and families around ethical concerns must do so.

Developing Guidelines

To start, the committee needs familiarity with current institutional policies and practices. Any current regulations or laws having a bearing on the policy under discussion should be reviewed. Professional standards should be included, as they relate to the issues at hand. Published protocols and advisory documents should be taken into consideration. The mission of the organization must be reflected in the policy, since it will be a statement of its values and beliefs. The committee developing these policies must support debate and differences of opinion. Reaching full consensus may take several years.

A policy on withholding and withdrawing treatment might contain the following components:

- A statement affirming the right of competent patients to make their own choices about treatment. Inherent in this belief is the concept of informed consent. The policy must affirm a patient's right to receive information about the various treatment options, their risks and benefits, and any particular information an individual patient might need to make an informed choice.
- Explanation about the components of informed decision making.
- A statement about the role of surrogate decision makers.
- Explanation about the role of assent in pediatric decision making.
- Explanation about the use of advance directives. Clarification of the state law, if any, should be included. However, recognition should be given to advance directives initiated in other states, since they are clearly the written wishes of a patient concerning healthcare decision making.
- A definition of Do Not Resuscitate orders, which would be helpful in eliminating confusion with partial code errors.
- Clarification about accepting or not accepting verbal or telephone orders for withholding or withdrawing treatment.
- Clarification that the order should clearly state the treatments that are to be withdrawn or withheld. For example, when a Do Not Resuscitate order is written, other treatments such as antibiotics and laboratory testing should be reviewed with the decision maker. It can be proper to discontinue some but not all treatments, since the comparative benefits and burdens may differ for different treatments.
- Clarification about the elements of documentation before a specific procedure is to be carried out. For example, such documentation might include but not be limited to discussions with the decision maker, other family members, and the healthcare team; the outcome of consultations with other professionals; and the supporting medical information.
- Explanation about the components of supportive care, particularly focusing on physical care, the presence of family or friends, pain management, and particular preferences of the patient.

- Clarification about who could or would withdraw the life-sustaining treatment. Nurses can withdraw the ventilator, yet they may want the physician present, or they may not want to be the one to withdraw the treatment. The institution should support either position.
- Clarification about a health professional's right to refuse to render care. This part should reflect the logistics of facilitating this refusal and the role of management.
- A statement on the organization approach to the resolution of disputes.

Implementing the Guidelines

Creation and adoption of a decision making policy does not guarantee acceptance or accurate implementation by the larger healthcare team. Once the guidelines are completed, provision for education, not just dissemination, must occur. Attending medical staff, resident staff, nursing staff, and other professional groups, as well as administration, must be included. Educational programs initiated before publication would help acceptance and quicker application of the concepts. In addition, the committee should develop a method for reviewing and revising them when necessary.

The hospital should maintain up-to-date resource material on bioethical issues and make it readily available to employees. Resources would include specific journals devoted to ethics, articles on specific topics that have been fully discussed by the committee, books focusing on current bioethical issues, information on court cases that have set precedents in the area of ethical decision making, and information on legislation that impacts how decisions are made within the healthcare institution. Working closely with a hospital librarian, if available, can facilitate this endeavor. Institutions wanting to establish effective and current guidelines must seek the knowledge to sustain them.

Summary

Guidelines define moral obligations in areas of conduct where the law may permit discretion or offers no direction. Guidelines set forth ideals of practice as well as clarify prohibitions. They establish a standard to be achieved rather than wrongs to be avoided. Guidelines facilitate communication and collaboration among the healthcare team. They are not a cookbook for ethical conduct; they are but a recipe that requires the incorporation of nuances in practice. In particular, a patient's preferences must guide the interventions. Most importantly, the existence of guidelines say to patients and families that a particular organization has the conviction and courage to establish moral norms that ensure proper deliberation and accountable decision making. Institutional policies should not be followed in a ritualistic manner. They do not become a new set of legalistic rules. They must continue to be open to discussion as changes occur in patient care and in society, and as healthcare professionals become adept in ethical decision making. An institutional ethics committee, nursing ethics council, and ethics education can support this endeavor.

REFERENCES

Fowler, M. D. M. (1988). Ethical guidelines. *Heart and Lung, 17*(1), 104.

In re Jobes, 210 N.J. super. 543, 510 A.2d 133 (super. Ct. Ch. Div.), review denied (N.J. Mar. 10, 1986).

In re Jobes, 108 N.J. 394, 529 A.2d 434 (1987).

Jameton, A. (1984). *Nursing practice; the ethical issues.* Englewood Cliffs, NJ: Prentice-Hall.

Joint Commission on Accreditation of Hospitals. (1987). New and revised standard approved: Withholding resuscitative service. *JCAH Perspectives, 5*(6), 5.

Longo, D. R., Warren, M., Roberts, J. S. & Dunlop, G. R. (1988). Extent of "do not resuscitate" policies varies across healthcare settings. *Health Progress, 69,* 66–73.

Smith, D. H., & Veatch R. M. (1987). *Guidelines on the termination of life-sustaining treatment and the care of the dying.* Indianapolis, IN: Indiana University Press.

8

The Allocation of Scarce Nursing Resources

Who will receive nursing services? How much care will they receive? On what basis will these decisions be made? Who will choose how a nurse spends her time? The answers to these questions appear more critical as the reality of the nursing shortage has become more evident. More registered nurses than ever are utilized in hospitals, the actual number of young people entering nursing is decreasing, and there is an attempt to replace the registered nurse at the bedside with less well-educated and more functionally oriented individuals. However, had the profession of nursing clarified firmly its position on these matters, had all nursing managers been clear in their utilization of the registered nurse, then the answers would not be so urgent. There has finally been a recognition that some of the recruitment and retention issues do involve increased dollars. However, this has come at a time when the hospital budget is being squeezed by both the payers for healthcare and the providers of all services. To fully appreciate nursing's dilemmas and opportunities within this environment, our discussion must initially focus on the economic picture for healthcare. We will examine the societal forces that have contributed to the increased dollars spent on healthcare services, the response of the federal government and other payers to this increase, and how society grapples with the dilemmas of who should get what, when. Finally, we will turn back to nursing and focus our attention on the realities at the bedside, and how the nurse manager can step in and initiate changes that will benefit individual practitioners and clients for years to come.

Healthcare Economy

Healthcare has become the nation's third largest business (Reinhardt, 1989). A successful business should be able to develop a profitable market share, based on competitive prices, excellent consumer relations, and unique items or services. These goals all contribute to a success that is ultimately measured in financial terms. However, healthcare institutions, particularly hospitals, are unique. Until recently, these above-mentioned goals have been pursued as ends unto themselves, unhampered by financial outcomes. Hospitals simply charged more when finances became tight. Currently, these goals are being severely threatened. Success is being measured by financial well-being, and efforts that contribute to this outcome are being rewarded.

A Historical Perspective

The economic picture for healthcare has become quite complex. Healthcare costs rose from 6.4% of the gross national product (GNP) in 1967 to 10.7% in 1983 (Gibson, Wando, & Levit, 1983). Despite intense efforts to control costs, healthcare expenditures continued to increase from 10.3% of the GNP in 1984 to 10.7% in 1986 (Rice, 1988). It is further anticipated that even with current economic controls to decrease costs, healthcare could consume 13.1% of the GNP by 1995 ("Health Care," 1989).

The late 1950s and early 1960s was a period of building and expansion in the healthcare industry, particularly for acute care hospitals. The enactment of the Hill-Burton Act provided monies to aid hospital industry growth. In exchange, hospitals agreed to treat a specified number of indigent patients free. The enactment of Medicare and Medicaid in the mid-1960s solidified an increasing social sensitivity in the United States to the aged and the poor.

Up until 1975, hospitals benefited from an increased utilization of hospital beds. This was due, in part, to advances in medical technology, an increased number of elderly and chronically ill individuals, and the growth of the insurance industry, which increased the availability of healthcare and effectively insulated the consumer and providers of healthcare from direct concern with cost. There was a belief that costs would go down as demand for service rose.

Until the mid-1970s, this belief continued, and funds were freely made available for treatment, education, and research. Most hospitals took their share of patients insured by governmental programs. Generally, individual and institutional providers believed it was their moral responsibility to treat all people who presented themselves for care.

However, the costs of healthcare grew beyond everyone's expectation. Techniques such as kidney dialysis, joint replacement, and coronary bypass surgery were extending life, relieving pain, and otherwise enhancing the quality of life, but at enormous costs. The rapid availability of advanced technology, coupled with a sicker population of patients, drove costs even higher.

By the mid-1970s, clear choices had to be made. A federal policy shift from one of open access to one of cost containment began to take hold. The overall payment mechanism remained that of cost-based reimbursement, but the federal government was asking hospitals for more financial controls to hold down costs. Hospitals reacted by proposing voluntary cost-control measures aimed at eliminating waste and inefficiency. However, strategies such as cutting back on supplies and conserving electricity had little effect on overall costs. These factors accounted for less of the problem than was realized. The harder issues relating to utilization patterns or outcomes of care, which may have provided information about efficacy of treatment and physician practice patterns, were not looked at. In fact, attention to these concerns did not occur for over 10 years.

As hospitals called for voluntary cost-cutting programs, businesses were instituting their own strategies. By 1983 businesses were seeing decreasing profits due to escalating healthcare spending. By 1986 over 200 business coalitions devoted to healthcare cost containment had been formed (Himmelstein & Woolhandler, 1988). Businesses, including hospitals, began to self-insure their employee health insurance programs in an effort to cut costs. Corporations forced providers to lower prices and shifted costs to employees through copayments and deductibles.

Prospective Payment

The early 1980s saw a more economically stringent approach to healthcare spending, as national health policy shifted from guaranteed access to cost containment. In 1983 a prospective payment system (PPS) for Medicare was instituted. It changed healthcare reimbursement from a cost-based retrospective system to a fixed-price prospective system. Medicare began to pay hospitals a preset price for services to its beneficiaries, based on average costs of hospital care for patients in diagnosis-related groups (DRGs). "Prospective payment is a system for packaging payment for services; therefore, a system of averaging. PPS averages historical costs, historical medical practices, and historical health care values" (Young, 1986).

The advent of prospective payment contributed to the proliferation of health maintenance organizations (HMOs) and preferred provider organizations (PPOs). Promising low costs for the consumer, HMOs and PPOs negotiated with hospitals for cuts in overall charges. By increasing competition for the already shrinking private sector payer, the sicker and more financially at-risk patients are being seen in public and university hospitals at an increasing rate. Therein lies one of the pitfalls of prospective payment. The disproportionate burden these institutions are bearing is not being adequately compensated by the prospective payment system. Hospitals that admit a high volume of low-severity patients have little incentive to be more cost efficient. They make money on these DRGs. However, hospitals that admit a high volume of very sick patients requiring complicated care often have costs that exceed the DRG dollar payment. They are unjustly penalized for serving this critical population.

The PPS system does provide a mechanism for enhanced payments for exceptionally costly cases or those that require more days in the hospital. These cases are called "outliers." But there are restrictions as to how many outliers a hospital can have, and the payment is less than what the system would pay if the patient was not considered an outlier. Thus very sick patients become outliers and account for many of the losses under prospective payment. There can be no doubt that incentives to limit hospital admissions may result in some patients being denied essential healthcare services. There is a belief that incorporation of a severity of illness scale into the prospective payment structure would decrease this inequity. "Overall, the lack of a severity of illness measure may have created a perverse social incentive: the desire on the part of hospitals to avoid the patients who need their services the most" (Evans, 1983).

Severity of Illness

Severity of illness criteria are individual patient factors that identify the acuity of care needed and that may therefore increase or decrease the resources consumed for an individual within a given DRG.

The DRGs take into account the principal diagnosis, types of procedures performed, presence of complications or co-morbid conditions, discharge status, and patient sex and age. The goal of the system is to reduce the variability in lengths of stay within each DRG and thus to contain the costs. In other words, patients within a particular DRG should consume, over a stipulated amount of time, about the same amount of resources, after accounting for the above differences.

However, use of length of stay as a surrogate for resource consumption is a major drawback of the DRG system. It is based on the premise that the acuity of patients always decreases significantly as discharge approaches. In modern-day healthcare this is not often the case, and the variables mentioned above are not always sufficiently sensitive to varying degrees of illness severity.

One of the earliest severity of illness scoring systems was developed by Susan Horn. She outlined seven patient dimensions that impact the amount of resources consumed by an individual patient (Horn, 1987).

- Stage of the principle diagnosis
- Complications of the principal condition
- Concurrent interacting conditions that affect the hospital course
- Dependency on hospital staff
- Extent of nonoperating room procedures
- Rate of response to therapy or rate of recovery
- Impairment remaining after therapy for the acute aspect of the hospitalization

Utilization of this severity of illness index in conjunction with DRGs has proven effective in producing more homogeneous resource consumption groups than DRGs alone. The DRGs were implemented on a presumption that costs within a particular grouping would fall within a predictable pattern. In fact, Horn's work and that of others' has shown this to not be true within many of the DRG categories (Dougherty, 1989, p. 7). Studies are showing that if severity of illness criteria were incorporated into the DRG system, payments per case would then reflect more adequately the services rendered. Since DRGs do not adequately account for severity of illness, the nursing care that patients receive or should receive is not appropriately compensated for within the prospective payment system.

Under prospective payment, there is an incentive to decrease the quality of service, so that the cost does not exceed the payment. Patients are being discharged sicker, with fewer patients being discharged directly home. There is a dearth of appropriate, quality institutions to successfully facilitate the transition from hospital to home (Heinz, 1986). Patients are returning home with technology considered just a few years ago to be appropriate only for the hospital setting. If severity of illness were better adjusted for, "the consequences of negative incentives in the present DRG prospective payment system, such as premature discharge, decreasing quality of care, dumping sicker patients, and the great difficulties of the specialty centers, could be mitigated" (Horn, 1986).

The Late 1980s

Since the introduction of prospective payment, hospital admissions have declined, 4% in 1984, 4.6% in 1986, and 0.6% in 1987 (Gallivant, 1988). Average length of stay also saw a decline, from 9.9 days in 1983 to 8.7 days in 1985 (Iglehart, 1986). As a result, occupancy rates also dropped from 72.7% in 1983 to 63.6% in 1985 (U.S. Department of Health and Human Services, 1985).

Most third-party insurers, including state and federal programs, began to stiffen requirements to control the demand for services. Authorization became necessary before certain services could be provided. Second opinions became mandatory for costly treatments. Incentives were provided to employees who chose less costly options for health insurance, and copayments and deductibles were increased. Additionally, active utilization management programs were instituted by third-party payers to assess the appropriateness of services and charges. A 1989 study by Hewitt Associates of 822 employer-sponsored medical plans showed the following conclusions: 70% of plans require cost sharing, 45% offer higher coverage for outpatient services, and 49% require preadmission testing ("Currents," 1989). In fact, health insurance premiums are up 20% to 40%, pressuring employers to scrutinize their benefit costs (Goldsmith, 1989). The American consumer is being asked to become very conscious of the costs of healthcare.

Meanwhile, the increasing need for long-term care facilities to absorb sicker and sicker patients, the growing number of high-technology patients receiving healthcare services in their homes, and the rising concerns over more and more people having limited access to health services leave room for doubting the full economic impact of prospective payment on the healthcare system. A recent Health and Human Services (HHS) study reported that over 31 million Americans are uninsured ("News at Deadline," 1989). This population includes those who do not qualify for various public programs, high-risk groups who cannot obtain insurance, and deliberately uninsured groups. The President's Commission for the Study of Ethical Problems in Medicine and Bioethical Research concluded in its 1983 report "that clients' ability to pay was a major block to obtaining health-care services." No major changes have occurred since that report was issued. In fact, access issues are becoming critical. The forces of advanced technology, decreased availability of healthcare, and increasing numbers of older and sicker patients are very real.

The 1980s ended with third-party reimbursement getting tighter, fewer physicians accepting governmental insurance, and equipment vendors and home nursing agencies refusing to serve patients insured by governmental programs. There is now a movement to develop a system similar to DRGs that would curtail payments to individual physicians. Perhaps this will facilitate closer cooperation between the hospital and its physicians. However, there have been no such strategies proposed to control the costs that are driven by the manufacturers and vendors of equipment, drugs, and supplies. The costs of research and development for new technology and new discoveries get passed on to the hospital, which gets squeezed in the middle when third-party payers limit payments for such care.

Prospective payment has definitely had an impact. Three hundred and sixty-three hospitals have closed since 1963 ("Chicago's 10," 1988). One thousand more acute care hospitals are expected to close during the 1990s. It is predicted that only a few regional hospitals will be treating trauma victims or operating as organ transplant centers in the 1990s (Mayer, 1989). Los Angeles County has had 12 of its 23 original trauma hospitals pull out of the trauma system since its inception in 1984, due to reimbursement problems (Freidman, 1989). Three hospitals have pulled out of the Chicago trauma network in the last 18 months ("News at Deadline," 1989, p. 26). The future will demonstrate the consequences of these results.

In the midst of all the confusion is the reality that the healthcare dollar has become a precious commodity, competing with other needed programs such as education, transportation, the environment, and the military budget. Since there is less and less money to go around, decisions have to be made about where the money is to go. What services should be paid for? Should some services not be paid for at all, or only be available for individuals with private insurance? Ultimately, who will make these decisions?

Allocation and Rationing

Allocation is a term used to describe a system that sets apart one thing for a specific purpose, according to a defined plan. Rationing means "to distribute or divide in an equitable manner" (*Webster's Third,* 1965). Allocation usually implies that decisions are made at some level away from the actual source of distribution, where the rationing would occur. To further explain these two concepts, Evans has utilized the distinctions of macro allocation, which deals with decisions at a public policy level, and micro allocation, which focuses on patients at the bedside. Hicks (1985) believes that there are basically three levels of decision making when allocating resources. System-wide allocation is the first level. The decisions made at this level are primarily public policy decisions. How many resources should be allocated for healthcare versus the environment, defense, or education is decided at the first level. In general, the concern at this level is how to maximize social welfare by allocating limited resources among competing sectors. What benefits can be achieved if one decision is made rather than another?

At Hick's (1985) second level, decisions are concerned with the allocation of resources among alternative users within a particular allocation area, for example, healthcare. These decisions focus on what proportion of the resources will be used for illness prevention, organ transplants, or outpatient care. These decisions might be made by insurance companies and those that decide priorities for research grants. The third level is concerned with the internal operations of a specific facility or service. The major concern at this level is with the financial viability of the institution. Does money go to pharmacy for a new program, or to the nursing department? Will money be targeted for the obstetrical area or to build a cancer center?

The healthcare arena has changed in ways that were not predicted. The explosion of technology and its accompanying costs, sicker and older patients needing more and more nursing care, and the AIDS epidemic are all factors that have contributed to the cost increases, despite reimbursement controls. The current nursing shortage has caused nursing salaries to rise, also impacting available dollars.

Scarcity means that resources are inadequate to serve all in need; somebody must do without, and somebody must decide who that will be. It no longer is a question of whether some services will not be provided, or that some patients may not receive certain services. The issue really is *who* will receive *what* and *who* is going to make those decisions. These are questions discussed under the principle of justice, particularly distributive justice.

Distributive Justice

Distributive justice is concerned with the allocation of goods and services, benefits and burdens, under conditions of scarcity. If everyone could have as much as he or she wanted of something distribution would not be an issue. Generally, the formal principle of justice holds that equals are treated equally and unequals unequally, in proportion to their relevant differences (Beauchamp & Childress, 1983). The significant question is on what basis does the distribution occur? What constitutes a relevant difference between people that would justify one person getting a resource instead of someone else? Several principles have been specified that attempt to identify just such relevant differences. These principles are termed "the material principles of justice" and have traditionally provided the basis for how scarce resources have been and are allocated in our society.

The material principles of justice assume that not all persons are equal for the purpose of distributing all of the goods and services in society. Therefore, relevant criteria must be defined to help determine on what basis resources are allocated:

- Distribution to each person according to effort or merit
- Distribution to each person according to societal contribution
- Distribution of an equal share to each person
- Distribution to each person according to need
- Distribution to each person according to free market exchange (Beauchamp & Childress, 1983)
- Similar treatment for similar cases (Outka, 1974)

Distribution According to Effort or Merit

Distribution of services based on effort and merit focuses on one's ability to expend energy to achieve a particular end. Utilizing these criteria is appropriate when granting college degrees, job promotions, and scientific awards. The criminal justice system appropriately hands out punishment based on merit.

However, in most healthcare situations, the allocation of goods and services based on merit or effort could be considered unjust and thus unfair. There are individuals in this society who, by age or disability, are unable to exert effort for individual achievement. Thus, the young and the old and those who are physically impaired or mentally handicapped would not qualify for a distribution of scarce resources just because they could not exert the same effort as others without these limitations.

The concept of effort also implies achieving health and thus meriting resources. Those who hold this view would argue that individuals who abuse alcohol and tobacco do not merit healthcare resources for illnesses that arise from these behaviors. Thus the smoker with chronic obstructive lung disease would not be admitted to the intensive care unit. Likewise, the alcoholic patient would not be eligible for a kidney transplant. Making decisions on this basis would also force healthcare providers to not admit the workaholic executive to the coronary care unit, or the race car driver to the emergency room after an accident. Certainly, all of these life-styles predispose one to a disproportionate share of health resources. Yet since smoking and alcoholism are more socially unacceptable, the natural tendency is to focus on individuals engaging in these habits.

Distribution Based on Social Contribution

For social contribution to be considered as a basis for distribution of healthcare services, the very young and the very old would be denied assistance. The young have not yet had an opportunity to contribute. The elderly, under this criterion, would not have any past contributions recognized. The negatively publicized dialysis committees of the 1950s used social worth as a criterion to assess a person's right to a dialysis machine.

Many of the characteristics that comprise individual differences and enable individuals to contribute to society are often based on luck or genetics. Therefore, the handicapped and the poor would be penalized with this type of criteria.

To Each an Equal Share

Central to the idea of distributing healthcare resources equally is the troubling question of whether healthcare is a right or a privilege. Although the phrase "right to health care" is frequently invoked, no such legal right has ever existed in the United States. Certainly, there is disagreement about whether Americans are due a certain level of healthcare, but except for emergency health service no such absolute right exists. To claim something as a right means that without it, an individual could be harmed. Because of this concern, most healthcare professionals, the general public, and the legislature agree that all individuals should be able to obtain some level of healthcare. However, this inclination is not matched by society's willingness to supply the financial resources necessary to provide the services. For example, some California hospitals refuse to serve patients paid for by the state's medical program, some physicians refuse to take Medicare assignments, and some hospitals, physicians, equipment vendors, and home health agencies refuse to serve Medicaid patients at all.

In other areas of governmental support, society has attempted to establish a minimum of service in the areas of education, housing, and transportation. Healthcare providers have been unable to answer the question of what constitutes the minimum services a person should receive so that he is not harmed if he does not get them. The trouble is that there is very little concurrence on what a decent minimum standard is.

Distribution to Each Person According to Free Market Exchange

Individuals with enough money would certainly benefit from this concept. This idea certainly is the basis for much of the inequity seen in the delivery of healthcare services. Every time the newspaper reports that a person was turned away from an emergency room due to inability to pay and subsequently died or was severely injured, the American public gets angry. When a family whose insurance will not cover an expensive treatment for their young child goes on television, the money pours in, and the hospital and doctors often donate their time. It is much easier for any society to make rules about abstract issues. It is another story when directly confronted with the outcomes. Most people do want to be just. "Like respect for persons, justice is so basic as to be nearly indefensible. In some ways, justice is a minimal claim on a social order. If we are to live among others according to rules of conduct, we should at least demand that these rules be fair" (Jameton, 1984).

Similar Treatment for Similar Cases

According to Outka (1974), this concept should guide our healthcare decisions. On the surface, the concept seems more than acceptable—it appears fair. Yet it still implies that everyone in similar circumstances gets the resources that he/she needs. There is simply not enough money to do this, particularly at the current rate of technological growth and the rise of debilitating chronic illness. Additionally, this scheme fails to define what need is. Outka admits that decisions where costs are prohibitive and situations where the "prospects for rehabilitation [are] remote" would not receive resources. Society has yet to make the determination of which cases are to not be treated but has begun to grapple with the concept.

In April 1989, the Oregon senate voted to ration healthcare to Medicaid recipients. This decision brought forth many comments as the plans unfolded. Healthcare priorities were established, and these were grouped in categories from 1 to 10, with group 10 being the ones with the highest priority. Oregon's present Medicaid budget would only include those priorities within group 10. Daniel Callahan, director of the Hastings Center, "praised the state for grappling with the inevitability of rationing . . . in a more coherent manner," while Arthur Caplan, director of the University of Minnesota's Center for Biomedical Ethics responded, "Any statement that proposes rationing only for the poor is inherently unfair" (Southwick, 1989). Inevitably, some decisions will have to be made. The question is, How will these decisions be made? The current economic crisis in healthcare is perpetuating other factors on which goods and services will be distributed.

Distribution to Each Person Based on Need

For nurses, need has been the sole criterion for determining a relevant difference between individuals requiring nursing services. "Advocating distribution on the basis of need, however, fails to take account of the facts that (1) need outstrips resources and (2) need is an infinitely expansible concept" (Fowler, 1989). The concept of need also implies that a person would be harmed if his/her needs were unmet. Is a little harm OK? By whose definition is a little harm understood? When discussing this view of allocation, many believe that an individual's basic needs should be met. Yet there has been no agreement on what constitutes basic needs. Daniel Callahan, in his book *Setting Limits: Medical Goals in an Aging Society* (1987), discusses his belief that comfort measures and palliative measures provided by nurses are due all sick individuals. The nursing profession must come to some agreement about what are minimal nursing care needs and come to some consensus about what constitutes comfort and palliative measures. No one else should be defining this. The Code for Nurses states that

> the nurse provides services with respect for human dignity and the uniqueness of the client, unrestricted by considerations of social or economic status, personal attributes, or the nature of the health problem. . . . The need for health care is universal, transcending all national, ethnic, racial, religious, cultural, political, educational, economic, developmental, personality, role, and sexual differences. Nursing care is delivered without prejudicial behavior. (American Nurses' Association, 1985).

Nursing, as a part of the healthcare received by patients, must determine its minimums for all patients, and limits for others. Who will receive nursing care? How much care will they receive? On what basis will these decisions be made? The choices must be guided by moral principles. Certainly, need, ability to pay, age, prognosis, physician request, and institution-directed criteria have all been used. The principle of justice implores us to use morally relevant criteria to make these determinations. Weighing perceived benefits and harms may help us view this more critically. However, we must define these benefits and harms in data meaningful to patients. Additionally, past cost-cutting decisions made in ancillary and support services are now impacting healthcare institutions more severely. There finally may be no one else to do it, including the nurse. Now, during the nursing shortage, when there are not enough nurses to provide nursing services, much less to fill in for other departments, the hospital is feeling the crunch much more severely.

Cost-Benefit Analysis

Since we are discussing healthcare resources from an economic perspective, another way to decide what resources ought to be paid for would be to utilize a cost-benefit analysis. Instead of looking at individual patient criteria, one could review the outcomes of care. In business a new program's viability usually rests with its potential to show a profit. From a healthcare perspective, one would analyze the benefit produced in relation to the dollars spent. Therefore, the consequences or outcomes of care would determine what decisions will be made. In healthcare, the studies focusing on the utilization of intensive care units are addressing the efficacy of care within those units. In other words, does the outcome of intensive care interventions justify the expense of the intensive care unit? The studies have been demonstrating some clear trends. For example, some data suggest that the benefits of admission to the critical care unit may be overestimated in patients with exacerbations of chronic, irreversible diagnoses such as congestive heart failure or chronic obstructive lung disease (Chassin, 1982; Cullen, Ferrara, Briggs, Walker, & Gilbert, 1976). Yet most studies are not comparing data across different units, which would give some information about different practice patterns or other variables that improve outcomes.

Although studies differ in their definition of benefit, medical morbidity and mortality data seem to demonstrate a common thread when evaluating the efficacy of intensive care. Certainly this traditional view of defining benefit in terms of morbidity does not account for any nursing benefit a patient might receive. This attitude has fostered (or been fostered by) the illusion that intensive care units are only for patients needing intense technology, but not for patients needing *just* intensive nursing care. The stance of insurance companies, in refusing to pay for 1:1 or 1:2 nursing care for patients who are not in an intensive care unit, only serves to compound the issue. There seems to be a total lack of recognition of the services nursing provides that are distinct from medical technology—services that are often beneficial even when the technology has proven futile. Interestingly, Knauss and colleagues (1986), while studying the efficacy of intensive care unit admissions, found that units with a more autonomous nursing staff and those with collegial relationships between nurses and physicians had improved mortality and morbidity statistics. Studies are underway within that research group to look at this outcome more closely.

Additionally, this limited view of what constitutes a benefit does not recognize how an individual patient might describe a benefit, such as relief from pain or perhaps time to make decisions. Not everyone places the same value on certain benefits. Some benefits may not be able to be quantified, such as decreased suffering. Finally, as many would agree, "The central problem with this method is that it excludes moral considerations that many people find crucial" (Veatch, 1988). Efficiency appears to be the primary motivator. It fails to account for ethical principles, such as autonomy or fidelity, and, certainly, the principle of justice.

The Allocation of Nursing Resources

Nurses as consumers should concern themselves with allocation decisions at all levels of distribution. However, nursing as a profession must focus attention and energy on the second level of allocation, as defined previously by Hicks (1985). The profession must be actively involved in legislative and other processes that influence decisions about healthcare program funding. But it is the individual nurse working in a particular institution who must focus on Hicks's third level of allocation, what each patient will receive. This is the area on which we well focus our attention. Some of the ways nurses are asked to distribute their service and some of the ways they ought to allocate themselves, as they attempt to meet individual patient needs and institutional demands, will be reviewed. Nursing managers in particular must play a significant role by ensuring adherence to accepted practice standards, as they decide the utilization of nurses within a particular facility. In a survey of 176 chief nursing executives of acute care hospitals in Minnesota, the most frequent dilemma noted was related to the use and distribution of nursing resources (Sietsema & Spradely, 1987). The stage will be set by first discussing the availability of nurses. Then, how a nurse ought to spend her time and prioritize care will be examined. Patient acuity and staffing mix will be approached from the position of nursing decision making. Admission and discharge criteria, utilization management measures, and quality assurance parameters all influence how a nurse spends her time.

The Availability of Nursing Resources

With the current reality of the nursing shortage, the availability of registered nurses has taken on a critical dimension. According to an

American Hospital Association survey (1988), the average registered nurse vacancy rate rose from 4.4% in 1983 to 11.3% in December 1987. The report of the Secretary's Commission on Nursing (1988) also found significant shortages in nursing homes and home health agencies. The American Association of Critical-Care Nurses has identified the need for over 125,000 additional critical care nurses to fill existing vacancies. They predict this need will double over the next 12 years (American Association of Critical-Care Nurses, 1980). This reported shortage exists in the midst of substantial reductions in hospital inpatient days and with over 80% of nurses employed in nursing.

Yet providing nursing care today has become a far more complex service than it was even 10 years ago. A rising patient acuity has certainly contributed to an increased demand for the registered nurse. In 1972 hospitals employed 50 nurses per 100 patients; by 1986 the figure had increased 82% to 91 nurses per 100 patients (American Hospital Association, 1988).

Some, like the American Medical Association, would solve the nursing resource crisis by adding a new person to the already complex pool of healthcare personnel: the registered care technologist (RCT), who, with a high school diploma and a few months of training, will be ready to carry out the doctor's orders (Chavigny, 1989). As the next discussion on the utilization of a nurse's time will show, more workers are not necessarily better, nor will they meet the patient care needs that are required.

The Allocation of Time

Nearly everyone has a thought on how a nurse should spend her time. The physician wants the nurse available to do things for him, hospital administrators want the nurse to work more productively, patients want the nurse to do what she is supposed to do and to be nice while doing it, and nursing management wants the nurse to just do it all and not complain. Most nurses try to meet all these expectations and usually leave their place of employment with feelings of having left things undone and of patients' needs being unmet.

Nurses are confronted with doctors' "orders" for care, patients' requests for services, the demands of the institution, and the nursing care prescribed by the nurse herself. With usually too many demands and not enough time, the nurse must make choices. The nurse must ration her care. How this will be done and who will decide are the critical issues facing nurses.

Professionals who believe in individualized patient care and autonomy for the practitioner often see these values getting lost amid bureaucratic decision making. On what basis does an individual institution establish its values? Is there a greater value placed on the completion of doctors' orders or on all patient care needs? Is care only defined by medical orders? Does the institution value nursing's different contributions? The answers will say a lot about the ultimate values the institution holds and how nurses are utilized within a particular facility.

"With roots in the military and religious systems of society, it is no wonder that hospitals and the medical and nursing professions view 'Doctor's Orders' as rules of law" (Manthey, 1989, p. 26). As Manthey writes, "They are actually requisitions for hospital resources to be allocated in particular ways for an individual patient" (p. 28). This view gives the nurse a rather interesting perspective and would make for stimulating conversation when discussion the allocation of a nurse's time. Certainly, the emphasis on nursing orders and individualized patient care plans supports this notion. It just seems that Manthey has been the first, at least in print, to admit it.

Another view in looking at nursing time focuses on the differentiation of non-nursing activities and non-nursing clinical activities. Certainly, most would agree that indirect care activities such as running for medications and supplies that have not been delivered, walking patients to their cars at discharge, stocking rooms, cleaning up the general area, calling other departments repeatedly to do something for the patient, arranging for repairs of broken equipment, getting late trays, and so forth, is not nursing care. These activities should be handled by support service personnel.

Nursing has also supported non-nursing clinical activities, such as those associated with respiratory therapy and physical therapy. In some hospitals, it may make economic sense to have nursing provide more of these nonnursing clinical activities. Often it takes a lot of nursing time to contact other services and negotiate the timing of complementary procedures. Nurses who have been in nursing over 15 years will remember that many of these activities were originally defined as nursing care. However, if a decision is made to have nursing take back some of these activities, such as changing ventilator settings and administering aerosol treatments, it must be done deliberately and with consciousness of the economic and noneconomic impact (Watson & Strasen, 1987).

Other traditional nursing activities are being seen as below the skill level of a registered nurse and thus accomplishable by others. For example, giving a bath, taking vital sings, or ambulating patients is being defined as menial work. It is not unusual for physicians and hospital administrators to express dismay at a "registered nurse" doing these things. Yet giving a bath allows the nurse time to assess her patient and to teach; taking vital signs includes understanding the rationale behind appropriate cuff size, checking the patient's previous values, and immediately repeating a value in question. Ambulating the patient is an opportunity to assess improvement in gait, strength, and respiratory effort and discuss activity limitations at home. This is the work of a registered nurse. Nursing has done a poor job of explaining that.

Why nursing has allowed itself to be devalued and looked on as nothing but a vehicle to carry out doctor's orders and perform a multitude of tasks is certainly beyond the scope of this book. This is a problem for the profession that impacts heavily on the allocation of nursing time.

If you are feeling that the things nurses do are attempting to be patched into the health delivery system, you may be right, and caution is needed as discussions occur about who will help the nurse and what these individuals will do. Yet there is no doubt that as costs squeeze the healthcare system from one end and the nursing shortage squeezes from the other, there will have to be a redistribution of the things nurses do. Other individuals will be needed to support the registered nurse. Nursing managers must reread the nursing shortage studies that have emphasized the desire of registered nurses to remain at the bedside. It is hoped that within our healthcare facilities, nursing management will give the recommendations of the Secretary's Commission on Nursing (1983, p. 19) serious consideration:

1. With the support of their governing bodies, administrators of health care delivery organizations should design and implement innovative, cost-effective staffing methods that provide non-clinical support services on a 24-hour, seven-day per week basis. Health professionals, including nurses and physicians, should be consulted in this effort. Examples of these new methods include job restructuring, utilization of support personnel, innovative scheduling plans, and the application of labor-saving technologies.

2. Administrators of health care delivery organizations should adequately staff clinical service departments so that patient care can be provided during off-hours without unnecessarily requiring nurses to provide clinical support functions. In addition, changes in the operation of clinical departments should be evaluated for their impact on the utilization of nursing resources.

Finally, the commission's report (1988) emphasizes what most nurses know: Substitution increases the overall demand for nurses and heightens the stress of the working environment. . . . The lack of support services lessens the time RNs can spend in direct patient care and contributes to excessive work loads and frequent overtime. Furthermore, these circumstances affect nurses' self-esteem as professionals and contribute to poor job satisfaction, high stress, and high turnover rates.

Prioritization of Care

Ultimately, when there is too much to do and not enough time to do it in, nurses are told to prioritize care. The prioritization of patient care rarely involves planning which activities not to do. Most nurses never consciously deal with work not completed. The image of patients not appropriately cared for fosters feelings of guilt, frustration, and, ultimately, anger. Nurses do not learn how or when to prioritize care in school or at the workplace. In fact, what ought to get done goes something like this: "The concept is that if a nurse does a good job 'prioritizing' somehow 11 hours worth of work will be done in 8 hours—in a appropriate manner, of course. This translates into no irate doctors, patients or relatives, plus good documentation and care planning and high QA scores" (Manthey, 1989).

Professional decision making involves looking at what needs to be done and the resources available and then making a conscious choice. Do the vital signs really need to be done every four hours? Does a full bath have to be given? Can the times of the medications be changed to when more resources will be available? Can physical therapy come and get the patient for treatment? Too often these things do not get looked at, because it is always easier to just do things than to think about not doing them. Thus the needed teaching, the complex dressing change, the quiet discussion about preoperative concerns, the altering of room assignments for a distraught family that needs privacy, and the phone call to a patient's faraway daughter are the activities that never happen or get done so poorly that no one should have bothered. Wouldn't it be a novel idea to actually develop systems to help the nurse prioritize the demands on her time, without the preconceived notion that nursing orders always come second or third or . . . Failure to assume any responsibility for the things done and not done is not the mark of a professional and endangers nursing's very existence.

Managers must plan with their nursing staff for such inevitabilities. There must be daily thought given to changing unnecessary of inefficient orders. Some nurses take care of these issues by using the care plan and Kardex for report. Thus the on-coming registered nurse can follow-up on needed changes and does not have to repeat unnecessary work or ineffective patient interventions.

Although no one would argue that the quality of nursing documentation today far surpasses that of 20 years ago, everyone would also agree that in some institutions, it is repetitive and time wasting. Changes can be made that will still satisfy the regulatory agencies and facilitate continuity of care. Flow sheets can help, as well as standardized care plans. Standards should be developed for the type and frequency of documentation, and computerized supports must be increased.

Patient Acuity

The average acuity of patients should be included in the budgeted full-time equivalents (FTEs) in terms of nursing hours per patient day (HPPD). However, not all hospitals do this. The budget from one year to another may just be rolled over, without reviewing whether the acuity data had changed. Additionally, if the acuity measurement does not accurately reflect the care needed, the required number of staff will not be sufficient. For example, if the acuity system does not take into account different levels of teaching needed, discharge planning, coordination of services, and adequate assessment time, there will not be enough nurses to do all necessary nursing care. Instead, the focus will be on tasks, particularly medial tasks that require little nursing intervention. Indeed, many administrators, as well as physicians, have chosen to view nursing as a series of tasks. Thus, as was seen in the previous section, it is easier to parcel out the duties of the nurse.

Staffing Mix

The nursing shortage has propelled the increase use of non-registered nurses at the bedside. Yet one cannot help but be concerned as again money enters into these decisions. The fact that a predominantly registered nurse staff is too costly is a myth that prevails. Wolf, Lesic, and Leak (1986) studied the costs of nursing care on two structurally identical medical-surgical units. The primary nursing unit's daily average costs, with mostly registered nurses, were less per patient day than the team nursing unit. Of course, there is no disagreement that on specific nursing units, the use of licensed vocational nurses (LVNs) or nurses' aides could be a significant adjunct to patient care and may be a reality with the shortage of registered nurses. But let us not substitute judgment for rhetoric. Decisions must be deliberate ones, with the entire nursing staff involved, making decisions about what is needed and when and determining what patients do need from the professional nurse. The aura of the budget has often driven nursing managers and nursing staff so far apart, one could doubt that they have the same concerns.

Admission and Discharge Criteria

One of the facts about working in a bureaucratic structure as a nurse is that the numbers of patients to be served are usually out of the control of nursing. Admission and discharge policies, which units patients get admitted to, and what time they are admitted are usually the function of physician preference and administrative contracts with third-party payers. But nursing managers can work with both groups to facilitate patient admission and discharge in a way to avoid delays and not impact heavily on scarce nursing resources.

Yet, unfortunately, most physicians and hospital administrators view the necessity of a hospital admission as a need for technology and/or close observation. Actually, it is the need for a registered nurse who operates the technology and does the observing. The American Association of Critical-Care Nurses advocates that admission/discharge criteria be based on patient acuity (intensity of nursing needs) and standards of nursing care. The association has addressed a number of criteria and, among them, has emphasized that the process used to determine such criteria "significantly affects the nature of care rendered and the use of limited resources to deliver that care" (American Association of Critical-Care Nurses, 1987).

Think about this scenario:

A tertiary medical center is experiencing a very high census, already 30 patients a day over the budget projections. A neighboring hospital experiences a major nursing strike, putting the first hospital in the position of taking the striking hospital's most critical patients. In the hopes that the strike will be settled soon, the tertiary center continues to try to do business as usual. This results in excessive overtime, a much higher use of temporary agency nurses, patients backed up in the emergency room waiting hours for a bed, and attending physicians being quite angry when they cannot admit a patient on a timely basis. Somehow, the nursing department is able to maintain safe nursing care, but after 4 days, the picture is looking more grim. The nursing administrator requests that elective surgery be canceled and that all the attending physicians be notified that both beds and nurses are becoming a scarce resource. The hospital gives its support, but for the next week, nursing administration is scapegoated as the perpetrator of the admission crisis. One doctor exclaims in frustration, "I cannot believe that you are affecting my practice." This hospital, like many, required clear policies about what to do when admissions become tight, whether it be for lack of beds and/or nurses. The administration of this hospital failed to recognize not only why patients are admitted to hospitals but also that effective admission and discharge policies require a collaborative effort of nurses, doctors, and hospital administrators.

Utilization Management

Some hospitals utilize criteria developed by an external company or consultant to assess whether services provided are appropriate, whether they should be provided in the hospital, and/or whether they meet criteria for a specialty service, such as rehabilitation. Sometimes these criteria are adopted without ensuring that they are pertinent for the individual institution, and rely heavily on a medical model for care. For example, a criterion that patients must receive physical therapy for a certain number of hours a day in order to be eligible for a rehabilitation unit overlooks the needs of some patients who may not be able to tolerate such intensity of therapy. It also overlooks the contributions other services make toward rehabilitative care, including nursing.

The utilization of intensive care units also falls under this category, since the need for medical technology often drives the criteria. Nursing managers, who serve on utilization review committees, must ensure that knowledgeable nurses are involved in setting these criteria.

Quality Assurance

Lacking a clear understanding of nursing's contribution to patient care and, ultimately, the institution's reputation for quality, administrators may make unreasonable demands on nursing management. They believe that significant cost reductions can occur without loss of quality. Some administrators do not care how their results are achieved. Others define quality by patient satisfaction questionnaires that focus on how promptly the nurse answers the call light and how courteous and pleasant the caregivers are.

The quality of nursing care has traditionally been measured by quality assurance activities within the department of nursing. The topics for auditing are often likened to the values of nursing administration or the criteria of regulatory agencies. Many of the indices used measure the adverse outcomes of care, like infection rates, falls, and medication errors. However, quality should be measured in positive terms. What should be looked at is information that could delineate what patient care outcomes are achieved because of the services provided by nursing. Studies such as these will help nursing determine what practices should continue and what practices should be modified or expanded. They will demonstrate what nursing interventions prevent iatrogenic complications. Consequences of hospitalization and illness, such as incontinence, skin breakdown, contracture, nosocomial infections, pain, and fatigue, are all within the influence of nurses. Finally, outcome data will prove that nurses do make a difference. Nursing managers can use the results of the data to guide staff education and individual nurse recognition.

The outcomes of preoperative, preprocedural, and discharge education must be correlated to length of stay, frequency of readmission, need for home support, and the overall outcome of a return to self-reliance, or ease of caretakers. The activities by nursing to provide such education and preparation may be targeted during short-sighted cost cutting unless outcome data are available to support the efficacy and value, both in human and economic terms, of these activities. Reporting of these data to consumer groups and the legislature would increase public understanding that nursing care not only makes a significant contribution to patient well-being but also is an essential service. When the Health Care Finance Authority (HCFA) begins to rate the quality of acute care hospitals, the quality of the nursing care should be high on its list. The DRG system provides the impetus for verifying the healthcare value of nursing and for documenting through research that nursing care leads to shorter lengths of stay and other patient benefits. Such documentation will ensure a different approach to the allocation of nursing services.

Costing Out Nursing Services

Traditionally, nursing services were not considered essential to the revenues of a hospital. The advent of prospective payment caused an intense look at the largest labor-intensive service in any hospital. Studies have revealed that nursing, far from being the major portion of hospital costs, is actually one of the biggest bargains in healthcare, representing approximately 11% to 18% of total hospital costs (Sandrick, 1985). Separating out the costs for nursing care can demonstrate economic accountability and provide additional proof that nursing care makes a difference in patient outcomes. "Hospitals can no longer be silent with the knowledge that nurses are the glue of the health-care system" (Sovie, 1987, p. 16). Nurses are the most viable representatives of what the hospital values and the image the patient is left with; yet, to quote from a good business adage, the quality of the product must be consistent with the price.

Summary

Although prospective payment is not the sole cause of the concerns about how limited healthcare resources should get distributed, the system has contributed to the dilemmas. "It increases the difficulty of shifting hospital costs to finance uncompensated care and it decreases hospitals' willingness to shoulder this burden in a more competitive environment" (Dougherty, 1989, p. 9). It must be remembered that the impetus for prospective payment came from a severe deficit in the availability of dollars for the Medicare budget. Medicare was established as a promise to the elderly that when they no longer worked and potentially could not afford medical care, the federal government would provide for needed services. A promise indeed, but one fraught with difficulties. At the time of Medicare's enactment, policymakers seemingly forgot that the 75 million individuals born between 1946 and 1964 would one day grow very old (Friedman, 1986).

Nurses have a moral responsibility to identify and resolve issues related to the allocation of scarce resources. How healthcare is distributed affects the public good, and benefiting the public good in matters of health is a moral obligation inherent in the social contract between nursing and society (American Nurses' Association, 1980). The Code for Nurses reinforces the concept of a social contract and the need for nursing involvement in resource allocation: "The nurse collaborates with members of the health professions and other citizens in prompting community and national efforts to meet the health needs of the public" (American Nurses' Association Committee on Ethics, 1985).

The allocation of nursing services involves the identification and selection of certain criteria for determining how nursing resources should be apportioned. Whether we allocate based on age, prognosis, need, or ability to pay depends on how benefit and burden are assessed. As Fry (1986) stated, this decision making is an ethical decision since it involves "the normative assessment of what constitutes benefit and what constitutes harm in terms of nursing services." Are justice and fairness to take priority over autonomy? Should the nurse's assessment of what is in the best interest of the patient guide the allocation of the nurse?

Benefits and harms, both immediate and long-term, must be taken into consideration. It may be difficult to weigh the utilitarian beliefs that guide many institutions against individual patient welfare, which guides many nurses. Nursing staff at all levels must be involved in reviewing these decisions. Some consensus in how nurses should be utilized will help ensure that patients do receive necessary nursing care.

Not only does the nurse manager's accountability for decision making extend into this realm, but also decisions made about the allocation of nursing resources set the precedent for nursing's position in the institution and its ability to deliver patient care. Nursing managers must pave the way for a definition of values that will guide nursing practice. Nursing must be on the front lines of any decision making efforts involving the allocation of nursing resources. Nurses themselves are best suited to make the decisions about how their services should be allocated.

Change is seldom comfortable. It is usually easier to go along with the group and make no waves. Yet the prospective healthcare system offers opportunities for nursing that must not go unexplored. How a nurse should spend her time and prioritize her services must be looked at when considering nursing's overall productivity. The acuity of patients should drive nursing's availability, not economically determined mixes. Quality assurance is an important tool to justify the contributions nursing makes; it must reflect outcomes of nursing intervention. Ultimately, utilization management programs and admission and discharge criteria will play significant roles in the allocation of all health services. Costing out nursing services will emphasize the significant economic contributions of nurses.

Nurse managers must work with staff to define priorities; help them utilize intershift report to review the nursing plan of care, as well as the medical orders; and help and support them in deciding that the order for vital signs is too frequent, changing an ineffective treatment that is being done just because it is written, and prioritizing care to facilitate a satisfactory discharge.

Pressures on healthcare professionals to contain costs threaten the delicate balance of needed patient care and cost-effectiveness. The conflicts for the practitioner are inevitable. The conflicts for the manager, the nurse manager in particular, are unavoidable. The ethical principle of autonomy received its heaviest applause in an atmosphere where doing more was becoming very costly. The increasing willingness to allow patients to exercise their autonomy in relation to withholding and withdrawing care does have some economic drivers. However, the importance of patient autonomy should not be underestimated, nor should it override all else. The balancing of autonomy and justice must occur between the policymakers and healthcare providers.

When costs must be decreased, it is too easy to decrease FTEs, decrease managerial layers, and give up secretarial support. Instead of cutting these areas, closer attention must be paid to reviewing the factors that get in the way of nursing productivity within an institutional context. This must be nursing management's direction for the future. The seeming enormity of the task and the multitude of variables must not undermine this focus. Managers must become knowledgeable in the facts and not be defeated by assumptions about the answers. Rather, a clear vision must be communicated. Nursing management may need to be the initiator of a joint effort of nursing, medicine, and hospital administration to understand the complexity and interrelatedness of the factors that influence the allocation of nursing resources.

REFERENCES

American Association of Critical-Care Nurses. (1980). Landmark study confirms the nursing shortage. *Administrative Chronicle, Fall.*

American Association of Critical-Care Nurses. (1987). Guidelines for admission discharge criteria in critical care. *Position Statement.* Newport Beach, CA.

American Hospital Association. (1988). *Draft report of the 1987 hospital nursing demand survey.* Chicago: Author.

American Nurses' Association. (1980). *Nursing: A social policy statement.* Kansas City, MO: Author.

American Nurses' Association Committee on Ethics. (1985). *Code for nurses with interpretive statements.* Kansas City, MO: American Nurses' Association.

Beauchamp, T. L., & Childress, J. F. (1983). *Principles of biomedical ethics* (2nd ed.). New York: Oxford University Press.

Beauchamp, T. L., & Childress, J. F. (1989). *Principles of biomedical ethics* (3rd ed.). New York: Oxford University Press.

Callahan, D. (1987). *Setting limits; medical goals in an aging society. New York: Simon & Schuster.*

Chassin, M. R. (1982). Costs and outcomes of medical intensive care. Medical Care, 20, 2.

Cavigny, K. H. (1989). Medicine vs. nursing, the RCT proposal. *Nursing Management, 20*(8), 38–40.

Chicago's 10 metro closures highlight urban-hospital fragility. (1988). *American Hospital Association News, 24,* 37.

Cullen, D. J., Ferrara, L. C., Briggs, B. A., Walker, P. F., & Gilbert, J. (1976). Survival, hospitalization changes, and followup results in critically ill patients. *New England Journal of Medicine, 294,* 982–987.

Currents. (1989). *Hospitals, 63,* 98.

Dougherty, C. J. (1989). Ethical perspectives on prospective payment. *The Hastings Center Report, 19,* 7, 9.

Evans, R. W. (1983) Health care technology and the inevitability of resource allocation and rationing decisions. Part II. *Journal of American Medical Association, 249,* 2208–2219.

Fowler, M. D. M. (1989). Biographic limits to life-extending technology. *Heart and Lung, 18,*(2) 204.

Friedman, E. (1986). 50 years of U.S. health care policy. *Hospitals, 60,* 102.

Friedman, G. (1989, July 31). Patient care not immune from cuts. *Healthweek*, p. 57.

Fry, S. T. (1986). Moral values and ethical decisions in a constrained economic environment. *Nursing Economics, 4*,(4), 161.

Gallivan, G. (1988). Margins drop, utilization improves in 1987. *Hospitals, 62*,40–42.

Gibson, R. M., Waldo, D. K., & Levit, K. R. (1983). National health expenditures. *Health Care Financing Review, 5*(1) 1–31.

Goldsmith, J. (1989). A radical prescription for hospitals. *Harvard Business Review*,67(3), 104.

Health care in the 1990s: Forecasts by top analysts. (1989). *Hospitals, 63*, 34.

Heinz, J. (1986). The effects of DRG's on patients. *Business and Health, July 8*,17–20.

Hicks, L. L. (1985). Using benefit-cost and cost-effectiveness analysis in health-care resource allocation. *Nursing Economics, 3*, 78–84.

Himmelstein, D., & Woolhandler, S. (1988). The corporate compromise: A marxist view of health maintenance organizations and prospective payment. *Annals of Internal Medicine, 109*, 494–501.

Horn, S.D., & Backofen, J. E. (1986). Ethical issues in the use of a prospective payment system: The issue of a severity of illness adjustment. *The Journal of Medicine and Philosophy, 12*, 150.

Iglehart, J. K. (1986). Early experience with prospective payment of hospitals. *New England Journal of Medicine, 314*(22), 1460–1464.

Jameton, A. (1984). *Nursing practice, the ethical issues.* Englewood Cliffs, Prentice-Hall.

Knauss, W. A., Draper, E. A., Wagner, D. P., & Zimmerman, J. E. (1986). An evaluation of outcome from intensive care in major medical centers. *Annals of Internal Medicine, 104*, 410–418.

Manthey, M. (1989). Just what are doctor's orders, anyway? *Nursing Management, 20*(1), 26.

Manthey, M. (1989). Who owns a staff nurse's time? *Nursing Management, 20*(9) 23–24.

Mayer, D. (1989, July 31). Hospital horoscope: More automation, fewer inpatients, *Health Week*, p. 22.

News at deadline. (1989). *Hospitals, 63*, 14.

Outka, G. (1974). Social justice and equal access to health care. *The Journal of Religious Ethics, 2*, 11–33.

President's Commission for the Study of Ethical Problems in Medicine and Bioethical Research. (1983). *Securing access to health care.* Washington, DC: US Government Printing Office.

Reinhardt, U. (1989). U.S. forces benefit/cost crisis in health care. *AHA News, 25*(24), 8.

Rice, D. P. (1988). Rationing care: The elderly are an easy target. *Hospitals, 62*, 26.

Sandrick, K. (1985). Pricing nursing services. *Hospitals, 59*(22), 75–78.

Secretary's Commission on Nursing. (1988). *Final report.* Washington, DC: Department of Health and Human Services.

Sietsema, M.R., & Spradely, B. W. (1987). Ethics and administrative decision-making. *Journal of Nursing Administration, 17*, 4.

Southwick, K. (1989, Apr. 17). Rationing moves ahead in Oregon. *Healthweek*, pp. 1–27.

Sovie, M. D. (1987). Exceptional executive leadership shapes nursing's future. *Nursing Economics, 5*(1), 16.

U.S. Department of Health and Human Services. (1985). *Report to Congress: The impact of the medicare hospital prospective payment system, 1984 annual report.* Washington, DC: Government Printing Office.

Veatch, R. M. (1988). Justice and the economics of terminal illness. *The Hastings Center Report, 18,* 36.

Watson, D., & Strasen, L. (1987). The integration of respiratory therapy into nursing. *Hospital & Health Services Administration, Aug.,* 369–377.

Webster's Third New International Dictionary. (1965). (3rd ed.). Springfield, MA: Merriam-Webster.

Wolf, G. A., Lesic, L. K., & Leak, A. G. (1986). Primary nursing: The impact on nursing costs within DRG's. *Journal of Nursing Administration, 16*(3), 9–11.

Young, D. (1986). PROPAC: Future directions. *Nursing Economics, 4,* 13.

SUGGESTED READINGS

American Hospital Association. (1987). *Surviving the nursing shortage strategies for recruitment and retention of hospital nurses.* Chicago: Author.

American Nurses' Association. (1985) *Code for nurses with interpretive statement.* Kansas City, MO: Author.

Applegate, M. L., & Entrekin, N. M. (1984). *Teaching ethics in nursing.* New York: National League for Nursing.

Beauchamp, T. L., & Childress, J. F. (1989) *Principles of biomedical ethics* (3rd ed.). New York: Oxford University Press.

Blanchard, K., & Peale, N. V. (1988). *The power of ethical management.* New York: William Morrow & Co.

Commission on Nursing Services. (1973). *Standards for nursing services.* Kansas City, MO: American Nurses' Association. Chicago: Author.

Davis, A. J., & Aroskar, M. A. (1983). *Ethical dilemmas and nursing practice.* (2nd ed.). Norwalk, CT: Appleton-Century-Crofts.

Fowler, M. D. M., & Levine-Ariff, J. (1987). *Ethics at the bedside: A source book for the critical-care nurse.* Philadelphia: J. B. Lippincott.

Jameton, A. (1984). *Nursing practice: The ethical issues.* Englewood Cliffs, NJ: Prentice-Hall.

Kohnke, M. F. (1982). *Advocacy: Risk and reality.* St. Louis: C. V. Mosby.

Report of the Special Committee on Biomedical Ethics. (1985). *Values in conflict: Resolving ethical issues in hospital care.* Chicago: American Hospital Association.

Ross, J. W, Bayley, S. C., Michel, V., & Pugh, D. (1986). *Handbook for hospital ethics committees.* Chicago: American Hospital Association.

Secretary's Commission on Nursing. (1988). *Final Report.* (Vol I). Washington, DC: Department of Health and Human Services.

Smith, D. H., & Veatch, R. M. (Eds.). (1987). *Guidlines on the termination of life-sustaining treatment and the care of the dying.* Indianapolis, IN: Indiana University Press.

Veatch, R. M., & Fry, S. T. (1987). *Case studies in nursing ethics.* Philadelphia: J. B. Lippincott.

INDEX

A
Accountability, 7–8, 26, 31–32, 70, 78
Accreditation, 66–68
Admission and discharge criteria, effect on resource allocation, 149–150
Advance directives, 30
Adverse reactions, 62
Advocacy, 2–8, 23, 64
  exploration of, in hiring interview, 12
  and institutional environment, 96–98
  and risk versus duty, 5–7
Allocation. *See also* Nursing resources, allocation of
  decision making about, 136–137
  definition of, 136
American College of Healthcare Executives, code of ethics, 64–65
American Medical Association, Code of Ethics, *See* Medical code of ethics
American Nurses' Association, 19
  Code for Nurses. *See* Code for Nurses
Autonomy, 3, 29–30
  and allocation of resources, 153
  and beneficence and nonmaleficence, 33
  individual nurse's, 31–32
  limits to, 30–31
  and nursing responsibility, 31

B
Beneficence, 32–36
Bioethical decisions, 28–29
Bioethics, 18, 50
Bureaucracy
  and ethical standards, 1–2
  and role conflicts for nurses, 2

C
Civil Rights Act of 1964, 92
Code for Nurses
  development of, 19–22
  and nurse manager's obligations, 10–11
  revisions of, 22–23
  on safe and ethical practice, 2, 4–5, 17, 19–23, 37, 39, 58, 64, 70, 74, 78, 86, 94, 125, 152
Code of ethics, 17. *See also* Code for Nurses; Medical code of ethics
Code of Hammurabi, 23–24
Communication, and safe and ethical practice, 11, 98, 118
Competence, 58
  and continuing education, 81
Confidentiality, and confronting unsafe practice, 77
Conscientious objection, 69–70
Consent. *See also* Informed consent
  valid, vs. informed consent, 31
Continuing education, in preventing unsafe practice, 80–81
Corporate culture, 8–9
Creativity, in safe and ethical practice environment, 12–13
Credentialing, 67–68

D
Diagnosis-related groups, 132–134
Disciplinary action, 38
Distributive justice, 137–143. *See also* Healthcare resources, distribution of
Do Not Resuscitate policies, 123
DRGs. *See* Diagnosis-related groups
Due care, 35

E
Education. *See* Continuing education; Ethics education
Employee support resources, 81
Ethical decision making, 4, 27, 41–60
  clinical case example, 54–57
  management case example, 57–60

Ethical decision making (*contd.*)
  model for, 45–46
    stages of, 46–52
    uses of, 53–60
  nurses' styles of, 41–42
Ethical dilemmas
  analyzing, 46–47
  causes of, 44–45
  definition of, 43
  in nursing, 43–45
Ethical environment, creating, 1
Ethical guidelines, 121–129
  development of, 126–128
  implementation of, 128
  institutional, 122–126
  resources on, 128
Ethical issues
  in health care, 101
  specific to nurses, 110–111
Ethical principles, 27–28
  and ethical decision making, 50–51
Ethics
  in clinical nursing practice, 2
  definition of, 1–2, 18
  descriptive, 18
  vs. morals, 18–19
  non-normative, 18
  normative, 18
Ethics education, 13–14, 117–118
Ethics rounds, 115–117

F
Family, involvement in ethical dilemmas, 48
Fidelity, 36
Florence Nightingale Pledge, 19–20, 39

G
Guidelines. *See* Ethical guidelines

H
Harm, 35
  and unsafe practice, 73
Healthcare, as right vs. privilege, 139
Healthcare costs, historical perspective on, 131–132
Healthcare economy, 131–136
  cost-control measures, 132
    effect on allocation of resources, 153–154
  historical perspective on, 131–132
  prospective payment, 132–134, 136, 152
  recent developments in, 135–136
Healthcare expenditures, historical perspective on, 131–132
Healthcare resources, distribution of
  according to free market exchange, 140
  according to merit, 138–139
  according to need, 141–142
  according to social contribution, 139
  cost-benefit analysis of, 142–143
  equality in, 139
  similar treatment for similar cases, 140–141
Health insurance, 135
Health maintenance organizations, 133
Hippocratic Oath, 24
Hiring interview, as opportunity to explore ethics and practice environment, 12
Hospitals
  and healthcare economy, 136
  legal responsibility, for quality of care, 66
  means for evaluating physician practice concerns, 76–77

I
Iatrogenic illness, 62
Impaired professional, 71–73
Incident reports, 66–67
Incompetent practice. *See also* Unsafe practice
  legal requirement for reporting, 65–66
Infant care review committee, 103
Informed consent, 3, 29–30
  and nursing responsibility, 31
Institutional ethics comittee, 102–110
  access to, 107
  advantages and disadvantages of

108–110
authority of, 108
case review by, 105–107
documentation by, 108
frequency of meetings, 108
functions of, 105
membership, 102–105
organization of, 107
quality assurance, 110
Institutional review board, 102

J
Justice, 76, 137, 140. *See also* Distributive justice
material principles of, 138

L
Law
and ethics, 49
and whistleblowing, 90
Leadership, in safe and ethical practice environment, 12–13
Legal consultation
about nursing dilemmas, 47
and whistleblowing, 91–92
Legal requirements, for reporting incompetent practice, 65–66
Loyalty, 4–5, 70, 86–87

M
Medical code of ethics, 23–26, 37
vs. Code for Nurses, 26–27
on professional responsibility for safe practice, 64
Medical ethics, education in, 117–118
Metaethics, 18
Mission statement, 8
Moral development, stages of, 42–43
Moral distress, 121
Moral reasoning, and moral action, 42
Moral uncertainty, 121

N
Narcotic records, audits, 72
National Labor Relations Act, 92
Negligence, by omission, 87
Nonmaleficence, 32–36
Nurse manager
and accountability issues, 32
and allocation of nursing resources, 153
and autonomy, 32
in facilitation of safe and ethical practice environment, 10–13
and professional ethics, 35–36
responsibility for confronting unsafe practice, 75–77, 81
and veracity, 38
Nurses, and institutional ethics committee, 104–105
Nursing ethics council, 110–115
advantages of, 115
case examples, 113–115
case presentation to, 112
members, 112–113
policies and guidelines formation by, 115
resources for establishing, 115
Nursing philosophy, 9–10
Nursing resources
allocation of, 130–154
criteria for, 152
nurses' involvement in, 152–153
availability of, 143–144
devaluation of, 146
time, allocation of, 144–147
Nursing services, costing out, 151

P
Patient acuity, and allocation of nursing resources, 148
Patient advocacy. *See* Advocacy
Patient care, prioritization of, 147–148
Patient safety, threats to, 85–86. *See also* Harm
Physician, concerns about unsafe practice by, confronting, 76–77
Policies and procedures, and unsafe practice, 79
Position statements, 121–122
Preferred provider organizations, 133
Professional associations
position statements by, 121–122
and whistleblowing, 93
Professional ethics, 17–40
fit with ethical thinking, 17
Professional values, 10

Prognosis committees, 102
Promises, 36
Prospective payment system, 132–134, 136, 152

Q
Quality assurance, 80
  and nursing care, 150–151

R
Rationing
  decision making about, 136–137
  definition of, 136
  of healthcare, 140
Refusal of treatment, 30
Registered care technologist, 144
Reprisals, for reporting unsafe practice, fear of, 71
Risk, 38–39
  to nurse
    and advocacy, 5–7
    and reporting of unsafe practice, 71
    and whistleblowing, 94
  versus responsibility, 6

S
Severity of illness, and healthcare resource allocation, 133–134
Staffing mix, and resource allocation, 148–149
Standards of care, 79–80
Substance abuse, among professionals, 71–73
Surrogate decision makers, 30

T
Technological imperative, 59
Termination, and whistleblowing, 92
Third-party reimbursement, 135–136
Treatment
  benefits and burdens of, 33–34
  withholding and withdrawing, policies on, 123, 125–128

U
Unsafe practice
  causes of, 68–70
  confronting, 73–75
    and institutional environment, 96–98
    nurses' professional responsibility in, 64
    and staff reactions, 78–79
  definition of, 62
  environmental factors in, 79–81
  legal requirements for reporting, 65–66
  organizational responses to, 77–79
  reporting, obstacles to, 70–73
Utilization management, effect on resource allocation, 150

V
Values, 43
Veracity, 36–38

W
Whistleblowers
  legal protection of, 92–93
  types of, 95
Whistleblowing, 71, 84–99
  approach to, 88–94
  consequences of, 94–96, 98
  definition of, 85
  procedure for, 93–94
  risks of, 94

HELP WANTED !

We would like your opinion of the CREATING AN ETHICAL ENVIRONMENT issue of Nurse Managers' Bookshelf :

____

____

____

Topics that you would like to see in future issues :

____

____

Name & Phone number (Optional)

____

____

Please mail to : Sue Glover, Williams & Wilkins
428 East Preston Street Baltimore, Maryland 21202
or, FAX TOLL FREE to Sue Glover 1-800-447-8438
THANK YOU FOR YOUR COMMENTS !

- -

☐ **YES !** Start my subscription to
Nurse Managers' Bookshelf (#6532-7)

_____ Individual Subscription $45.00 (4 Issues)
_____ Institutional Subscription $60.00

I am also interested in ordering the following back issues at $19.95 each (or all four for $45.00):
_____ Recruitment & Retention
_____ Communicating Like a Manager
_____ Performance Evaluation
_____ Team Building

❑ Check Enclosed ❑ Bill Me ❑ Master Card ❑ VISA ❑ Amex.

Card#______________________________ Exp. Date__________

Signature or P.O.#______________________________

Name ______________________________

Address ______________________________

Mail to Williams & Wilkins P.O. Box 1496 Baltimore Md. 21298-9724
Call TOLL FREE from anywhere in the US 1-800-638-0672
or FAX 1-800-447-8438